SpringerBriefs in Public Health

T0172148

SpringerBriefs in Public Health present concise summaries of cutting-edge research and practical applications from across the entire field of public health, with contributions from medicine, bioethics, health economics, public policy, biostatistics, and sociology.

The focus of the series is to highlight current topics in public health of interest to a global audience, including health care policy; social determinants of health; health issues in developing countries; new research methods; chronic and infectious disease epidemics; and innovative health interventions.

Featuring compact volumes of 50 to 125 pages, the series covers a range of content from professional to academic. Possible volumes in the series may consist of timely reports of state-of-the art analytical techniques, reports from the field, snapshots of hot and/or emerging topics, elaborated theses, literature reviews, and in-depth case studies. Both solicited and unsolicited manuscripts are considered for publication in this series.

Briefs are published as part of Springer's eBook collection, with millions of users worldwide. In addition, Briefs are available for individual print and electronic purchase.

Briefs are characterized by fast, global electronic dissemination, standard publishing contracts, easy-to-use manuscript preparation and formatting guidelines, and expedited production schedules. We aim for publication 8–12 weeks after acceptance.

More information about this series at http://www.springer.com/series/10138

Jeffrey S. Markowitz

Mortality Among Hispanic and African-American Players After Desegregation in Major League Baseball

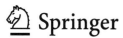 Springer

Jeffrey S. Markowitz
Health Data Analytics
Princeton Junction, NJ, USA

ISSN 2192-3698   ISSN 2192-3701   (electronic)
SpringerBriefs in Public Health
ISBN 978-3-030-17279-4   ISBN 978-3-030-17280-0   (eBook)
https://doi.org/10.1007/978-3-030-17280-0

This Springer imprint is published by the registered company Springer Nature Switzerland AG
The registered company address is: Gewerbestrasse 11, 6330 Cham, Switzerland

Preface

Growing up in an Epicenter

In the mid-1950s, I was a young boy growing up in Brooklyn, less than 5 miles from Ebbets Field, the home of the Brooklyn Dodgers. The train ride to Ebbets Field cost 15 cents and took about 20 min. As I would understand years later, I was growing up near the epicenter of baseball's "Great Experiment" (Tygiel 2008) of reintegrating African-Americans into Major League Baseball after more than a half-century hiatus. Known as "Dem Bums," a nickname derived from a complicated mix of fans' affection and derision, most Brooklynites, like myself and my friends, loved the Dodgers. As I saw things, even at my youthful age, there were two major obstacles constantly confronting Dem Bums: the New York Giants, the inter-borough, intra-league rivals who played at the Polo Grounds in upper Manhattan, and the New York Yankees, the "Bombers" from the Bronx.

Most of us fiercely disliked the Giants as they had a knack of preventing the Dodgers from getting into the World Series. Perhaps, the best-known example of this occurred in 1951 when the Giants beat the Dodgers on a home run in the bottom of the ninth inning in the final game of their National League playoff series to advance to the World Series. Russ Hodges' famous radio call of the home run hit by Bobby Thompson—also known as "the shot heard round the world"—that won the game and the National League pennant for the Giants that afternoon added insult to injury for Dodger fans. With uncontrollable glee, Hodges shouted repeatedly: "the Giants win the pennant, the Giants win the pennant...." a total of 5 times. Though too young to recall this tragic moment, I have encountered stark reminders hundreds of times throughout my life.

As much as my friends and I disliked the Giants, it was the New York Yankees that most Dodger fans truly despised. Playing their home games at Yankee Stadium, the so-called "house that [Babe] Ruth built," the Yankees were the gold standard in baseball. Between 1921 and 1959, the Yankees appeared in 24 World Series and won 18 of them. In comparison, the Dodgers played in a total of eight World Series during this same period and won just two of these. And guess who beat the Dodgers in these six World Series losses? If you guessed the Yankees, unfortunately, you are correct. It was an intense, lopsided, bitter, intra-city rivalry that New York City baseball fans cherished year after year.

While the Yankees dominated the Dodgers with respect to winning and losing baseball games, it was the Dodgers who led the way in desegregating Major League Baseball. Of course, this wasn't a competition or anything, but in 1947, Jackie Robinson, playing for the Brooklyn Dodgers, became the first African-American to play in the Major Leagues since before the turn of the twentieth century. (It took the Yankees another 8 years to field their first African-American player, Elston Howard, in 1955.) To this day, I'm proud that the Dodgers were the first team to end the ugly scourge that was the Major League Baseball's color barrier. Putting aside "beating the Yankees" at something, the signing of Jackie Robinson by the Dodgers was a great source of pride to me and many others living in Brooklyn.

Jackie Robinson proved to be an outstanding baseball player during his 10-year Major League career, leading the Dodgers to their first World Series victory ever—beating the Yankees in 1955. Of far more importance, Robinson and the end of segregation in Major League Baseball helped to change the course of US race relations, and even US history. Several writers and historians believe that Robinson's entry into Major League Baseball served as the impetus for the US Civil Rights movement in the 1960s (Constitutional Rights Foundation 2018; Craig 2017).

My own love for baseball and its history was rooted in these Brooklyn years and has endured throughout my life.

My Uncles' Influence

Two uncles on my mother's side of the family, also Brooklyn residents, often came together to visit our family. During these visits, all my uncles wanted to do was watch baseball on our tiny black and white 21-inch TV. Though not many games were televised in the mid-1950s, my uncles always managed to appear for visits on days when there were games on TV, and exactly at the time when the first pitch would be thrown. Like my parents, both uncles struggled to make ends meet. In my parents' case, financial woes left them with little time or energy to develop an interest in baseball.

My uncles clearly adored the Dodgers, but also showed considerable interest in several non-Dodger players of the time like Roberto Clemente, Orlando Cepeda, Luis Aparicio, Minnie Minoso, and others. As I would learn years later, these were some of greatest baseball players of all-time, all born in Latin American countries. But why did my uncles care so much about baseball, in general, and these players specifically? As the years passed, and I better understood my uncles' backgrounds, I began to appreciate their fervor for baseball and their special interest in Latin American players. Both uncles had been born and raised in Havana, Cuba during the 1920s and 1930s where baseball had become very popular. (Both my parents also grew up in Cuba but were born in Poland.)

While baseball originated in the US, Cuba was the first Latin American country where the game was played. Baseball had become part of Cuba's national identity as they fought to gain their independence from Spain during the latter part of the nineteenth century. For many Cubans, baseball was a nationalistic treasure, an alternative to Spanish bullfighting, and a valuable part of their newly found independence. It was the Cubans who organized the first Latin American baseball league, and who helped spread baseball to other Latin American countries. To this day, baseball remains an integral part of Cuban life and culture, and like the US, baseball, rather than soccer, is Cuba's proud national pastime.

During the first half of the twentieth century, when African-Americans were banned from baseball, several Latin American players appeared on Major League Baseball rosters. Not only did these players have to be very talented, but their skin color had to be something other than black. Coinciding with the end of baseball's color line in 1947, Latin American players, even ones with dark skin color and visible African ancestry, began appearing in larger numbers on Major League Baseball rosters.

Curious About the Past

Baseball was, and still is, a sociocultural phenomenon with a complicated history. Combined with my uncles' influence, growing up at "Ground Zero" of baseball's integration piqued an evolving curiosity about the game and its players. This interest grew stronger as I progressed through high school, undergraduate, and graduate school.

Growing up in a Northeastern US city that was supposed to be relatively tolerant of racial and ethnic minorities, I can assure you that African-Americans as well as Hispanics faced racism and discrimination on and off the baseball field. I witnessed this on the streets of Brooklyn as well as at Dodger games. I saw first-hand how Jackie Robinson and other African-American players that followed him into the League were treated by some white players, coaches, and fans. I saw the bean-balling and the spiking and heard the racial epithets. These unfortunate realities of that time have been documented in more than a few books (Zeiler 2013; Ruck 2011; Moore 2011; Lamb 2012; Tygiel 2008; Rust Jr 1992; Burgos Jr 2007). "The larger history—of racial struggle in Brooklyn and America after World War II —is often ugly and painful" (Sokol 2015).

As a Public Health student at Columbia University in New York City in the 1980s, I asked myself questions about race, national origin, and how this could impact on health. I knew that baseball was a statistics-crazy sport and believed that it might be possible to collect data on this subject. However, there was no Internet then and the available data on players' health and mortality was scanty. But now, nearly 40 years later, with an enormous amount of verifiable data on the Internet, the aging of players from the time of integration, plus decades of personal experience as an epidemiologist, I've decided to return to earlier questions from my youth and study the connection between race/Hispanic origin and mortality among former Major League Baseball players—specifically, by studying former players who played during the 40-year period after segregation had ended in the Majors.

Studying Death and Its Fairness

For many, the concept of death may be difficult to consider and I'm no exception. It's been painful to examine the deaths of many of my childhood heroes. Before writing this book, my previous (third) book titled "Mortality and its risk factors among professional athletes: A comparison between former NBA and NFL players" (Markowitz 2018) focused on comparing mortality risk between two professional groups of former players. Altogether, I've been studying mortality for about 5–6 years now. The death of most professional athletes, including Major League Baseball players, is generally a public matter, particularly when a player is a star, dies young, or has a nonnatural cause of death. Despite the certainty of death, hearing about the passing away of a former player always surprises me. It's hard to fathom how strong, remarkable athletes can succumb to anything—even death.

Nevertheless, the study of death can tell us much about life, perhaps even help to extend life in a quality manner for future generations. The study of special groups, like professional ballplayers, who may differ from their general population counterparts in terms of income, body size, and athleticism may also provide important preventative clues. Consequently, the study of death is indispensable to public health. Hence, while saddened when hearing about a players' passing, I feel fortunate to have the opportunity to study mortality among former ballplayers, many of whom I watched play and admired for years.

Several things about death that make it amenable for epidemiological study is that, with advancing age especially, it occurs in relatively large numbers, and there's variability with respect to when it occurs. In addition, while sometimes cruel and unexpected, there's nothing random about death from a statistical perspective.

Readers should rest assured that this is not a philosophy book, but a fundamental question related to mortality has to do with its *fairness*. Putting aside issues related to pain and suffering, I think most would agree that death affecting the elderly disproportionately more than the young seems "fair." There are also gender differences in life expectancy. As the "life expectancy champions" (Zarulli et al. 2017), females currently live longer than males in the US as well as almost every place else in the world (Barford et al. 2006). This is largely due to biological, genetic, social, and environmental factors. This may seem unfair (especially if you're a guy), but since it's a worldwide phenomenon and the factors advantaging females are largely immutable, many (including myself) will accept their longer longevity as being fair.

However, is it equitable that whites in the US tend to live longer than African-Americans? When one considers the possible man-made reasons for these differences, such as education, income, access to quality health care, and discrimination, it becomes hard to justify the fairness of between-race mortality differences that advantage one group over another. Moreover, many public health and government officials agree with me on this matter. In 1990, for example, the US Department of Health and Human Services issued its Healthy People 2000 initiative (CDC 2009), which promoted a comprehensive strategic plan for improving health in the US by the year 2000. This plan contained hundreds of health-related goals and objectives including the need "… to address the overreaching goal of reducing health disparities in special populations at higher risk than the total population for death, disease, or disability" (National Center for Health Statistics 2001). Some specific objectives of the plan focused on *reducing* mortality-related disparities that disadvantaged African-Americans. By 2010, the goals of the Healthy People 2020 initiative focused on *eliminating* rather than reducing health disparities, and for 2020, 1 of 4 overarching goals of Healthy People 2030 was to "achieve health equity, eliminate disparities, and improve the health of all groups" (CDC 2011).

The sad fact is that mortality differences based on race have been documented in the US general population since records have been kept. But do such disparities have to continue, and what can be learned from special groups like former professional athletes to help reduce or eliminate between-race mortality differences? Does Hispanic origin play a role in mortality risk among former Major League Baseball players including those who played during the post-segregation era? These and other important questions will be addressed in this book.

Brief Overview of this Book

This book studies mortality and mortality risk among more than 5200 former Major League Baseball players. Individuals who participated in the league as players anytime between 1947, the year that baseball desegregated, and 1986 will be studied. Most of this cohort, about 80%, is non-Hispanic whites, and certainly there are many great men and outstanding baseball players within this group. Without diminishing the contributions to the game made by former non-Hispanic white players, the significance of the roughly 1000 African-American and Hispanic individuals who played Major League Baseball during the post-segregation years cannot be overstated. By all accounts, many of these players endured ridicule, scorn, and other indignities from fans, the media, playing opponents, and teammates. Many African-Americans were subject to discrimination before, during and even after their baseball playing careers had concluded. In many ways, Major League Baseball was (and may still be) a reflection of the broader US culture which in some circles embraces racism as a way of life.

Many of the African-American and Latin American players who played Major League Baseball following the end of segregation were trailblazers and heroes with numerous books and other publications describing how these players overcame poverty, little or no education, difficult living situations and other adverse circumstances to play professional baseball (Zeiler 2013; Ruck 2011; Moore 2011; Lamb 2012; Tygiel 2008; Rust Jr 1992; Burgos Jr 2007). With the passage of time, the aging of these 1000 African-American and Hispanic players has now also made it possible to examine another important part of their story—their mortality.

Some individuals who played Major League Baseball in the late 1940s could have been born during the first decade of the twentieth century, and, predictably, most of these players have now passed away. In addition, players born in the 1920s (and later) may have already passed away too. Given the roughly 1000 African-American and Latin American players who participated in Major League Baseball during the post-segregation period (up to the year 1986) and their advancing ages as of 2018, it has now become feasible to statistically analyze comparative mortality among these groups of players based on their race and national origin. While the vital status of these African-American and Hispanic players is the focus of this book, there were also more than 4200 non-Hispanic white players who played Major League Baseball between 1947 and 1986 who are obviously a vital part of the story as well, and their mortality statistics become critical for purposes of comparison.

Before delving into the empirical study that's the focus of this book, it's essential to examine the history and evolution of professional baseball in both the US and Latin America. Chapter 1 contains a brief history of baseball as well as its social and cultural underpinnings in the US. The roots of baseball cannot be fully separated from several critical historical events in the US like the Civil War and Reconstruction. The end of the Civil War led to the abolition of slavery. Yet despite Constitutional amendments passed between 1865 and 1870 that were supposed to help equalize rights between the races, discrimination and racism persisted. Jim Crow laws and court rulings during the first part of twentieth century continued to foster an uneven culture that favored whites over African-Americans, particularly those residing in the Southern part of the US.

Chapter 2 offers a very brief history of Latin America that is centered on those countries that have contributed players to Major League Baseball during the years following the end of segregation. Like the US, Latin America was colonized by Europeans who sought to use slave labor as the basis of their economies. Before the slavery would end, a very racially and ethnically mixed culture would evolve in Latin America comprised of various combinations of indigenous people, Europeans and Africans. Baseball, essentially an import from the US, first arrived in Cuba and then became popular in several other Latin American countries.

For more than a century now, US general population mortality statistics consistently indicate that African-Americans are disadvantaged mortality-wise compared to whites. The literature and statistical review described in Chap. 3 documents these inequalities based on data published by the Centers for Disease Control and Prevention (CDC). Not only is there a long-standing gap in life expectancy between the races, but overall death rates as well as death rates for heart disease and cancer are consistently higher among African-Americans. The CDC statistics also indicate that Hispanics residing in the US have better mortality statistics than African-Americans, and often fare better than non-Hispanic whites. However, statistics can sometimes be complicated and this "Hispanic Paradox"— the idea that Hispanics living in the US tend to have equal or better mortality outcomes relative to non-Hispanic whites despite being disadvantaged socioeconomically—warrants closer scrutiny.

The empirical analysis begins in Chap. 4 with a description of the methods and the study hypotheses. Based on the literature review provided in Chap. 3, many readers will anticipate mortality predictions for African-American players relative to their non-Hispanic white counterparts. In contrast, given the uncertain state of mortality patterns among Hispanics, hypotheses related to comparisons between former Major League Baseball players from Latin American countries will be more difficult to formulate.

Chapter 5 presents basic descriptive statistics for key study variables like race/Hispanic origin, year of birth, and vital status. Simple cross-tabulations of vital status by race/Hispanic origin are given that are stratified by year of birth categories. Very preliminary testing of the study hypotheses will be described in Chap. 6. The goal of the analyses described in Chaps. 7 and 8 will be to identify other variables that could be important in understanding the relationship between race/Hispanic origin and mortality within the study cohort. As will be shown, there are several other variables besides race/Hispanic origin—such as educational attainment (Chap. 7), body mass index (Chap. 8, Sect. 8.2), US birthplace region (Chap. 8, Sect. 8.4) number of career years played Major League Baseball (Chap. 8, Sect. 8.6), player position (Chap. 8, Sect. 8.8), and handedness (Chap. 8, Sect. 8.10) —that may be statistically related to either or both race/Hispanic origin as well as mortality. The question then becomes whether these items add *independently* to the prediction of mortality as risk or protective factors, and/or change the statistical association between race/Hispanic origin and mortality. Multivariate independent predictors of mortality will be uncovered in Chap. 9. Within the boundaries of the variables included in this study, this multivariate analysis will serve as the definitive test of whether race/Hispanic origin is a risk factor for mortality among the former Major League Baseball players who played in the era following desegregation.

Up to this point in the book, all the empirical analyses are "internal" since they are restricted to players in the study cohort. Chapter 10 is an "external" analysis because it compares mortality rates observed among cohort players to the US general population, matched for age, gender, and race. Standardized Mortality Ratios (SMRs) will be generated for each race/Hispanic origin group using US Census data answering the question whether mortality rates are higher, lower, or about the same between the three groups of professional athletes and their general population counterparts. Chapter 11 will offer my perspective on what the study findings mean and where we go from here in terms of future research needs. Study limitations will also be discussed.

Delving into race and mortality disparities that exist more broadly in the US general population will not be the easiest or most comfortable matter to discuss. Yet, in the context of this pressing public health issue, a dialogue is needed to further unravel the causes of disparities and what can be done to reduce them.

Ground Rules

Use of Player Names
Player names will be used sparingly and only in chapters that do not contain empirical analyses. As many baseball and other sports fans know, there's a wealth of demographic and player-related information published online and in hundreds of sports books and publications. Nevertheless, details related to player lives and deaths could be sensitive material for surviving family members, friends, and fans, especially when this information is presented in complex ways involving combinations of variables that, heretofore, have not been made public. Out of respect for research privacy rules and policies like those published by HIPAA, or Health Insurance Portability and Accounting, (US Department of Health and Human Services 2003) player names will *not* be included within the empirical chapters of this book.

References to Race and Hispanic Origin
The main independent variable in this study is race/Hispanic origin. Players born in the US are divided into two racial groups, African-Americans and non-Hispanic whites. The third group consists of players born in Latin America. I have chosen to use the term "African-Americans" in this book. Other authors quoted in this book have used other terms and expressions which may include "Blacks," "Black Americans," and "Afro-Americans." In some cases, these terms can be used interchangeably, although others have different meanings. In my writing, I attempt to help readers better understand what is meant by other authors when they use different words to describe various racial and ethnic groups.

My decision to use "Hispanics" rather than "Latinos" was a difficult one to make since the use of both words has pros and cons. The main factor for me in deciding to use "Hispanics" is that it's used by many others cited in this book including government organizations and authors. For example, I often sourced general population data on "Hispanics" published by the CDC and refer to the "Hispanic Paradox" dozens of times. Although I prefer Latino as the more empowering term from a cultural and historical perspective, using Hispanic is more consistent with the relevant literature.

For purposes of this book, Major League Baseball players born in the US who are not African-American are white. Moreover, because we also know that they were not born in a Latin American country, these players will be called "non-Hispanic whites." Based on an analysis of Hispanic surnames (Word and Perkins 1996), there are only about a dozen US players in the cohort who come from Hispanic backgrounds, and while not perfect, these players will be aggregated with the non-Hispanic white players. To summarize, the 3 groups that are the focus of this book are African-Americans, non-Hispanic whites, and Hispanics. The name I'll use to describe this grouping variable will be "race/Hispanic origin."

Other authors may use alternative words and terms to describe various races or other combinations of race and national origin. When this occurs, the authors' words and terms will be noted and used in the text and table displays.

The Need for Solid Statistics

This is a research study that examines specific hypotheses related to how mortality risk may be related to the race/Hispanic origin of former Major League Baseball players. In addition, strategies are used to rule out alternative explanations. Consequently, the approach is based on sound statistical methods and techniques. While many readers may be interested in the subject matters covered in this book, some will not have the statistical background necessary to understand the analyses presented in Chaps. 6–10. In these chapters, an attempt is made to explain statistical matters to accommodate a broad range of readers. To this end, each empirical chapter concludes with a "Summary of Empirical Results" section that will detail, in nontechnical terms, the statistical conclusions that have been reached. Also, readers interested in nonstatistical explanations of results should look for sentences that begin with the phrases "In other words…." or "This means…"

It may be difficult to "enjoy" a book that focuses on mortality. This is particularly true when the deceased includes individuals who many see as sports heroes. So instead of saying that I hope readers enjoy this book, my goal is that you find it interesting, informative, and meaningful. As a public health professional, my primary objective is to help extend quantity and improve quality of life, particularly for those with the greatest need.

Princeton Junction, NJ, USA   Jeffrey S. Markowitz

References

Barford, A., Dorling, D., Davey Smith, G., & Shaw, M. (2006). Life expectancy: Women now on top everywhere. *BMJ, 332*(7545), 808.

Burgos A., Jr. (2007). *Playing America's game: Baseball, Latinos, and the color line.* Berkeley: University of California Press.

CDC, Centers for Disease Control and Prevention. (2009). *Healthy People 2000.* Retrieved from https://www.cdc.gov/nchs/healthy_people/hp2000.htm.

CDC, Centers for Disease Control and Prevention. (2011). *Healthy People 2020.* Retrieved from https://www.cdc.gov/nchs/healthy_people/hp2020.htm.

Constitutional Rights Foundation. (2018). Jackie Robinson: Desegregation begins with baseball. Retrieved from http://www.crf-usa.org/black-history-month/jackie-robinson.

Craig, M. (2017). Baseball's integration and the contemporary civil rights movement. Retrieved from https://www.beyondtheboxscore.com/2017/9/25/16356568/jackie-robinson-integration-civil-rights-movement-jesse-owens-sean-doolittle-bruce-maxwell-racism.

National Center for Health Statistics. (2001). *Healthy People 2000 Final Review*, Hyattsville, Public Health Service. Retrieved from https://www.cdc.gov/nchs/data/hp2000/hp2k01.pdf.

Lamb, C. (2012). *Conspiracy of silence: Sportswriters and the long campaign to desegregate baseball*. Omaha: University of Nebraska Press.

Markowitz, J. S. (2018). *Mortality and its risk factors among professional athletes: A comparison between former NBA and NFL players*. Cham: Springer Nature.

Moore, J. T. (1988). *Larry Doby: The struggle of the American League's first Black player*. Mineola: Dover Publications, Inc.

Ruck, R. (2011). *Raceball: How the Major Leagues colonized the Black and Latin game*. Boston: Beacon Press.

Rust A., Jr. (1992). *Get that Nigger off the field: An oral history of Black ballplayers from the Negro Leagues to the present*. New York: Delacorte Press.

Sokol, J. (2015). Jackie Robinson's life was no home run for racial progress. *Time*. Retrieved from http://time.com/3942084/jackie-robinson-racial-progress/.

Tygiel, J. (2008). *Baseball's great experiment*. New York: Oxford University Press.

US Department of Health and Human Services. (2003). OCR HIPAA Privacy, Research. Retrieved from https://www.hhs.gov/sites/default/files/ocr/privacy/hipaa/understanding/special/research/research.pdf.

Word, D. L., & Perkins C., Jr. (1996). Building a Spanish surname list for the 1990s—a new approach to an old problem, Technical Working Paper No. 13. Retrieved from https://www.census.gov/population/documentation/twpno13.pdf.

Zarulli, V., Barthold Jones, J. A., Oksuzyan, A., Lindahl-Jacobsen, R., Christensen, K., & Vaupel, J. W. (2017). Women live longer than men even during severe famines and epidemics. Retrieved from http://www.pnas.org/content/pnas/early/2018/01/03/1701535115.full.pdf.

Zeiler, T. W. (2013). *Jackie Robinson and race in America*. Boston: Bedford/St. Martin's.

Acknowledgments

Many thanks to my dear wife and long-time academic partner, Dr. Elane Gutterman, Ph.D., for her outstanding editing as well as her many thoughtful suggestions for the content of this book.

Contents

List of Figures

List of Tables

Part I
The Backstory

Chapter 1
The Roots of Baseball in the US

1.1 Baseball in the US

Dating the origins of baseball depends largely on how one defines "baseball" (Vaught 2013). Ball and bat games can be traced back several millenniums to possible origins in Egypt around 1500 B.C. Fast forwarding 2500 years, ball and bat games were played in England following the Norman Invasion in 1066 (Vaught 2013). Remotely resembling baseball, a combination of 2 English games, rounders and cricket, was observed in the US during the eighteenth century (History Staff 2013). However, these early games had few similarities to baseball as it began to be played in the mid-nineteenth century.

Myths about the origins of modern baseball in the US are not uncommon. Baseball historians unanimously agree that the game was *not* invented by Abner Doubleday in Cooperstown, New York in 1839, as some business officials wanted fans to believe. In fact, Doubleday, a decorated Civil War Union Army General, was proclaimed the inventor of baseball as a nationalistic ploy at a meeting of Spalding marketing executives held in 1907 (McDonald 2016). The truth is that Doubleday never had anything to do with the game of baseball (History Staff 2013).

The patriotic facade of baseball was based on an American longing to have a sport that was native-born and raised—not imported from Europe or elsewhere. Thought by many to be a democratizing game, baseball would become, and still is, the national pastime in the US. In 1889, Mark Twain described baseball as "… the very symbol, the outward and visible expression of the drive, the push, the rush and struggle of the raging, tearing, booming nineteenth century" (Twain 1889).

During the early and mid-nineteenth century, baseball in the US was a social activity played by men as a form of leisure. In those days, fielders would get a runner out by "plugging" or "soaking" him, which meant throwing and hitting baserunners with the hard ball. The new so-called Knickerbocker Rules (Thorn 2004) did away with plugging which in turn helped reduced arguing and violence on the playing field (Baseball Reference 2018). In addition to tagging baserunners, or having the

© The Author(s), under exclusive license to Springer Nature Switzerland AG 2019
J. S. Markowitz, *Mortality Among Hispanic and African-American Players After Desegregation in Major League Baseball*, SpringerBriefs in Public Health,
https://doi.org/10.1007/978-3-030-17280-0_1

ball beat them to a base, the Knickerbocker Rules contained additional elements of baseball as played today, such as 90 feet between bases within a diamond-shaped infield, playing teams comprised of 9 players, foul lines, a 3-strike rule, and games that were generally 9 innings in length.

The first baseball team in the US in 1845, the New York Knickerbockers, was comprised of amateurs from an upper-class New York City Social Club (Thorn no date). Their first game in 1846, was played against a cricket team (History Staff 2013). Other baseball clubs emerged during this period, often along racial and ethnic lines (Ashe Jr. 1988). Initially, baseball was played mainly in the Northeastern US, although Civil War soldiers, who played the game in-between battles, helped spread the game throughout the country (Ruck 2011).

By 1857, there were 16 New York City area teams that formed the first amateur baseball organization, the National Association of Base Ball Players, or NABBP (Wright 2000). As the governing body of baseball, the NABBP organized the first championship games. By 1865, there were about 100 NABBP baseball teams and within the next 2 years, the number of teams quadrupled. While some star players were secretly paid for playing the game in the early days of the sport, baseball teams were primarily comprised of individuals who did not receive any compensation.

This changed in 1869 when 12 teams from the NABBP announced that they would turn professional. In 1871, the NABBP was replaced by a professional baseball league known as the National Association of Professional Base Ball Players, often called the National Association. In 1876, the National Association was replaced by the National League. The American League of Professional Baseball Clubs, later known as the American League, was formed in 1901 as the National League's rival. Two years later, the winners of the National and American Leagues competed in the first World Series. While many changes to the organization and structure of Major League Baseball have occurred since the beginning of the twentieth century, these are the same National and American Leagues that compete today.

1.2 African-Americans and Slavery in the US

The well-established issues that provoked the Civil War included states' rights, trade, tariffs, and especially slavery. Because baseball in the US took root before, during and after the Civil War, a brief account of slavery in the US is relevant.

In 1619, the first captive Africans were brought to Jamestown, Virginia by the Dutch and the degrading practices of slavery became prevalent in all US colonies. As a cheap and abundant source of labor, slaves worked mainly on large plantations or small farms, producing tobacco, indigo, rice, and cotton (after the invention of the cotton gin in 1793). By the time the African slave trade was outlawed in 1808, more than 400,000 slaves had been brought to the US. Despite this, a domestic slave trade persisted, resulting in a dramatic increase in the number of slaves. By 1860, it's estimated that about 4 million slaves resided in the US with about half in Southern states that produced cotton (History.com a no date).

Because of poor nutrition, impoverished living conditions, and dangerous work, slaves suffered disproportionately from a variety of conditions and diseases (Downs 2012). Sometimes referred to as "Negro diseases," these conditions included tetanus, cholera, tuberculosis, influenza, hepatitis and syphilis (Kiple and King 1981). When slaves became sick, their treatment was minimal, if not altogether absent. Not unexpectedly, slaves had short life expectancies. Only 4 of every 100 slaves in the US lived to 60 years of age or older (Frederick Douglass Family Initiatives 2018).

1.3   African-Americans in Baseball

Prior to the turn of the twentieth century, there were isolated periods when whites and African-Americans played organized baseball together. However, up until the time of Jackie Robinson's appearance in 1947, baseball in the US was a largely segregated game. With few exceptions, integrated baseball was only played in the more tolerant sections of the US, i.e., the Northeast and Midwest. The end of the Civil War and Reconstruction generated monumental hardships for African-Americans, particularly in the South. Nevertheless, organized amateur baseball became popular in the immediate aftermath of the war. During the next 20 years, roughly 200 all-African-American teams were organized throughout the country (PBS 2014).

According to the Baseball Reference history section: "As early as 1867, the racism of the post-Civil War era showed up in the national pastime: The National Association of Baseball Players … voted to exclude any club that had black players from playing with them" (Baseball Reference 2018). This period also saw the rise of Jim Crow laws in the US (especially in the South), which segregated the 2 races in most aspects of living and "… forbade whites and Blacks [from] competing in the same athletic contests" (Tygiel 1983). By 1872, with the disbandment of the NABBP, several African-American players appeared on the heretofore all white teams and became the first blacks in professional baseball. Several African-Americans played professional baseball together with whites during the 1870s and 1880s. However, [African-American players] "… were shunned by teammates, vilified by spectators, and brutalized by opponents" (Lamb 2012).

It was not uncommon for African-Americans to be targets of physically abusive play by white players during the games they played together. For example, white pitchers would sometimes intentionally throw balls at African-American batters' heads (McKissack and McKissack 1994; White 1907), a practice known as "bean-balling." The intentional spiking of African-American infielders by white baserunners also became a frequent practice in the integrated games. It was an act of self-protection when 2 of the first African-American professional baseball players, Bud Fowler and Frank Grant, both infielders, invented shin guards to help minimize injury when intentionally spiked by white players sliding into bases (Peterson 1970).

In the late nineteenth century, some white players engaged in practices to remove African-Americans from professional baseball games. For example, at an exhibition game in 1883, Cap Anson, a white player/manager for the Chicago White Stockings, and a future Hall of Famer, refused to take the field if the African-American catcher for the Toledo team was permitted to play. Again in 1887, Anson demanded that 2 African-American players on the opposing Newark team not be allowed to play in a scheduled game. Almost immediately after Anson's refusal to play against African-American players in 1887, directors of the International League, a vital Minor League baseball organization, "… decided that since white players had misgivings about blacks and had threatened to leave the league if something was not done, no more contracts would be offered to black ball players" (McKissack and McKissack 1994).

With no contract signings of African-Americans in baseball's Minor League system, blacks were phased out of Major League Baseball. By the end of the 1880s only a few African-Americans were playing Minor League baseball (Tygiel 1983). While never officially written, Major League Baseball's color line was codified by a policy known as the "Gentleman's Agreement" which effectively banned African-Americans from the game. Even the Commissioner of baseball, a former US federal judge named Kenesaw Mountain Landis, never acknowledged an official ban of African-Americans players in the League (Gurevitz 2015). Given the subterfuge in establishing Major League Baseball's color line, its start date is thought to be around 1892.

Although slavery had been abolished in the US and Constitutional amendments passed promising equal rights, African-Americans were barred from the country's national sport. Only with the introduction of Jackie Robinson into Major League Baseball in 1947 would the color barrier come to an end.

1.4   Baseball and the Larger American Society

During the years immediately following the Civil War there was a glimmer of hope "… that baseball—like America—could achieve its promise of equality for all" (Burgos Jr. 2007). After all, slavery had been abolished and amendments to the Constitution had provided African-Americans with citizenship, equal protection, due process, as well as the right to vote. Unfortunately, this legitimacy turned out to be more theoretical than real, particularly in the Southern part of the US, due to laws and policies that were intimidating and segregating. Even the US Supreme Court played a leading role in maintaining separation between African-Americans and whites. The infamous Plessy v. Ferguson Supreme Court ruling of 1896 legalized the doctrine of "separate but equal" (Legal Information Institute no date). While the "separate" part of this ruling was extolled by many whites, the "equal" part was either ignored or minimized by other rules and policies that ensured inequality for African-Americans.

After their forced removal from the Major Leagues, African-American professional players participated on predominantly black teams in organized baseball games. Perhaps the most famous of these teams, the Cuban Giants, was initially formed in 1885. Remarkably, several of the all- or predominantly- African-American teams were named "Cubans." This was intended to fool some opponents and fans into thinking that the players were Cuban rather than African-American. It has even been reported that "… [Cuban Giants] players chatted [Spanish] gibberish on the field to pass as Cubans" (Tygiel 1983).

African-American baseball teams during this period were plagued by unfair financial agreements. "Gate receipts were tightly controlled by white booking agents. The agents dictated when and where black teams could play, and they subsequently passed little of the games' attendance revenues on to team owners" (Kelly no date). In part, the frustration that arose from the unfair financial treatment of African-American owners and players, motivated Rube Foster, the "father of Black baseball" and a future Hall of Famer, to form the Negro Major League in Kansas City, Missouri in 1920.

Branching out from the Midwest, at least 7 Negro Leagues emerged in the East and the South in both urban and rural areas. Negro League baseball teams often participated in "barnstorming" games, traveling throughout the country and Latin America to play non-league games for pay. Negro League teams often played day games and traveled at night. As the financial pressures of Negro League players and owners intensified, some teams played both day and night games on the same day, even in different cities.

Because Negro League teams rarely owned their own stadiums, they rented venues from Major and Minor League teams. This money often represented a significant percentage of income for these organizations. For example, the New York Yankees alone made about $100,000 per year based on revenues from Negro League baseball (Bradbury 2007). Despite this, African-American baseball players were often not permitted to use the regular (all-white) locker rooms and showers. In addition, Negro League games were sometimes cancelled at the last minute by the Major and Minor League organizations when they were offered more lucrative situations.

By the 1930s, some of the greatest baseball players of all-time played in Negro Leagues. Nevertheless, it is generally accepted that the overall quality of Major League Baseball play was better than the Negro Leagues. Several African-Americans superstar players, like Satchel Paige and Josh Gibson, earned salaries that eclipsed those of most white baseball players. On average, however, the salaries earned by Major League Baseball players, exceeded those earned by Negro League players. According to one author: "… most [African-American] players earned between $125 and $300 a month, less than half the average white athlete" (Tygiel 1983). Many African-American players also played baseball during the winter months in professional leagues in Latin American countries. Notably, average salaries for Negro League baseball players exceeded those earned by African-Americans in the general population (Tygiel 1983).

1.5   The Role of World War II

Some writers and historians viewed the oppression of Jews in Europe as partly analogous to the situation experienced by African-Americans in the US. In many ways, American involvement in World War II was paradoxical: while the US was fighting for freedom and equality abroad, many African-Americans were denied these same basic rights at home. Just several weeks after the Japanese attack on Pearl Harbor, the Pittsburgh Courier launched the "Double V" campaign—victory in the war being fought against the Axis powers, plus victory at home in the fight against racism and inequality.

The Double V campaign encouraged African-Americans to serve in the US Armed Services during World War II and simultaneously called on them to demand implementation of the 3 post-Civil War equal rights amendments. The Double V campaign sought to fight fascism in Europe as well as racism, segregation and unequal rights in the US.

As in the broader US society, Jim Crow laws were pervasive in the military during the war. Although African Americans could volunteer for military service and even be drafted, when permitted to serve, they were relegated to segregated units and usually given menial jobs. "The world's greatest democracy fought the world's greatest racist with a segregated army" (Ambrose 1997).

Prior to World War II, less than 4000 African-Americans served in the US Armed Forces and there were hardly any African-American officers. By the end of the war in 1945, over a million African-Americans had served in the military with many integral to fighting and winning the war. Several segregated all- African-American military units were nationally acclaimed. For example, the Tuskegee Airmen flew more than 15,000 sorties in North Africa, Sicily and Europe and distinguished themselves as courageous, world-class airmen (Manning 2012). World War II had laid the groundwork for ending segregation in Major League Baseball.

1.6 Desegregation in Major League Baseball

Many social, political and economic forces impacted the battle over African-Americans' re-entry into Major League Baseball, and by the 1930s, the pressures to desegregate had intensified. The movement to integrate baseball was led by a variety of individuals and groups that included African-American and progressive journalists, white activists and civil rights groups. The movement occurred around the same time that other anti-discrimination struggles were underway related to housing, jobs, and education (Dreier 2013).

With the extensive involvement of African-Americans in World War II, tensions related to desegregating baseball increased in the 1940s. Clearly, many African-American baseball players were talented enough to play in the Major Leagues and many of them were already stars in Negro Leagues. Ostensibly, talented African-American players would improve the chances of Major League teams to win games, and perhaps even championships. Of most importance for some, ending segregation in Major League Baseball was the "morally right thing to do." While the separate but equal doctrine created by the Plessy v. Ferguson case dominated US race culture and policy, significant exceptions in the sports world had already become evident. For example, African-Americans represented the US at the 1932 and 1936 Olympic games and successfully participated in numerous college sports, like baseball and football.

Yet, some Major and Minor League baseball team owners feared that the Negro Leagues would not survive if African-Americans were permitted to play Major League Baseball. Unsubstantiated warnings were circulated around baseball that racial incidents would occur if African-Americans were permitted to play in the Majors. Moreover, there were more than a few Major League Baseball team owners, other executives and players who had anti-African-American feelings and beliefs. For example, one team owner, Tom Yawkey, grew up on a large plantation in South Carolina and strongly opposed the idea of ending segregation in Major League Baseball. His team, the Boston Red Sox, became the last to sign an African-American to a Major League Baseball contract (Kepner 2017), 12 years after Jackie Robinson broke the color line.

1.7   Jackie Robinson and the Desegregation of Baseball

Jackie Robinson, the grandson of a slave, was born on January 31, 1919 in a plantation shack in Cairo, Georgia. Jackie, the youngest of 5 children, was only a year old when his father left the family. Robinson's mother moved the family to Pasadena, California, where she worked a variety of jobs to sustain her family. As a child and young man in both Cairo and Pasadena, Robinson and his family faced numerous incidents involving segregation and discrimination (Tygiel 1983).

Robinson excelled at multiple sports in high school and college including football, baseball, tennis and track. Prior to being drafted into a segregated US Army unit in 1942, he played semi-pro football. Robinson went to Officer Training School, a rare feat for an African-American at the time, and in 1943, he became a 2nd Lieutenant in the US Army. However, Robinson's military career ended abruptly the next year following a racial incident when he was ordered, but refused, to move to the back of an Army bus. Court martial proceedings ensued on charges of "insubordination during questioning." Despite his acquittal, the Army would not allow Robinson to deploy overseas. Several months later, Robinson was honorably discharged.

In 1945, Robinson was offered a contract to play baseball professionally in the Negro League. Following 5 months of play for the Kansas City Monarchs, Robinson was signed to a contact with the Montreal Royals of the Brooklyn Dodgers' Minor League organization. The primary engineer of Robinson's ascent to Major League Baseball was Dodgers' team President and General Manager, Branch Rickey, a former college baseball coach. It is believed that Rickey was motivated to integrate baseball both morally, based on incidents he experienced while coaching, as well as economically. As part of the Great Migration, beginning around 1916 and continuing through 1970, about 6 million African-Americans transplanted themselves from Jim Crow dominated regions in the rural South to Northern, Midwestern and Western cities (Wilkerson 2016). As African-Americans populated large cities outside the South, many were known to watch and enjoy Negro League baseball. Thus, Rickey believed that signing Robinson would increase Dodger ticket sales. Rickey also felt that Robinson's participation would improve the team and perhaps help the Dodgers win a championship, a feat that had eluded the team since their inception in 1883.

During his 10-year career with the Dodgers, Robinson led the team to 6 National League pennants as well as their first World Series championship title in 1955. Inducted into the Baseball Hall of Fame during his first year of eligibility in 1962, the League also retired his jersey number 42 from all Major League Baseball, the only number to be honored in this manner. [Robinson's] "… dignified courage in the face of virulent racism—from jeers and insults to beanballs, hate mail, and death threats—commanded the admiration of whites as well as blacks and foreshadowed the tactics that the 1960s Civil Rights Movement would develop into the theory and practice of nonviolence" (History.com b no date).

Jackie Robinson died in October 1972 at the age of 53 from heart disease and diabetes complications.

The genesis and early development of professional baseball in the US coincided with massive political and cultural changes that fostered between-race inequalities that would persist for decades. Legal attempts to resolve these matters often met with resistance that made progress slow and difficult. African-American service during World War II was part of a social and political movement that helped set the stage for desegregating Major League Baseball. Rather than ending between-race inequalities, including health and mortality disparities, desegregation in baseball set in motion new changes and challenges. Hispanics also entered the US professional baseball fray in earnest beginning in 1947 with an influx of players that continues robustly today. A brief account of Latin American history, particularly as it relates to race and social class, follows in Chap. 2.

References

Ambrose, S. E. (1997). *Citizen soldier. The US Army from the Normandy beaches to the bulge to the surrender of Germany*. New York: Simon & Schuster.

Ashe, A., Jr. (1988). *A hard road to glory: Baseball*. New York: Amistad Press Inc.

Baseball Reference (2018): *History of baseball in the United States*. Retrieved from https://www.baseball-reference.com/bullpen/History_of_baseball_in_the_United_States.

Burgos, A., Jr. (2007). *Playing America's game: Baseball, Latinos, and the color line*. Berkeley: University of California Press.

Bradbury, J. C. (2007). *The baseball economist: The real game exposed*. New York: Penguin Group.

Downs, J. (2012). *Sick from freedom: African-American illness and suffering during the Civil War and Reconstruction*. New York: Oxford University Press.

Dreier, P. (2013). The real story of baseball's integration that you won't see in 42. *The Atlantic*. Retrieved from https://www.theatlantic.com/entertainment/archive/2013/04/the-real-story-of-baseballs-integration-that-you-wont-see-in-i-42-i/274886/.

Frederick Douglass Family Initiatives. (2018). Additional facts provided by the Gilder Lehrman Institute of American History. Retrieved from http://www.fdfi.org/additional-facts.html.

Gurevitz, A. E. (2015). Breaking Baseball's color line. *Arizona Journal of Interdisciplinary Studies, 4*, 86–101.

History.com a. (no date). Slavery in America. Retrieved from https://www.history.com/topics/black-history/slavery.

History.com b (no date). Jackie Robinson. Retrieved from https://www.history.com/topics/black-history/jackie-robinson.

History Staff. (2013). *Who invented baseball?* Retrieved from https://www.history.com/news/ask-history/who-invented-baseball.

Kelly, M. (no date). The Negro National League is founded. *National Baseball Hall of Fame.* Retrieved from https://baseballhall.org/discover-more/stories/inside-pitch/negro-national-league-is-founded.

Kepner, T. (2017). Thomas Yawkey, the Red Sox owner who resisted integration. *New York Times.* Retrieved from https://www.nytimes.com/2017/08/18/sports/baseball/red-sox-thomas-yawkey-integration.html?_r=0.

Kiple, K. F., & King, V. H. (1981). *Another dimension to the black diaspora.* UK: Cambridge University Press.

Lamb, C. (2012). *Conspiracy of silence: Sportswriters and the long campaign to desegregate baseball.* Lincoln: University of Nebraska Press.

Legal Information Institute. (no date). Plessy v. Ferguson. Retrieved from https://www.law.cornell.edu/supremecourt/text/163/537.

Manning, R. (2012). The 'Tuskegee Experiment': The legend of the Tuskegee Airmen. Retrieved from http://www.malmstrom.af.mil/News/Features/Display/Article/349719/the-tuskegee-experiment-the-legend-of-the-tuskegee-airmen/.

McKissack, P. C., & McKissack, F., Jr. (1994). *Black diamond: The story of the Negro baseball Leagues.* New York: Scholastic Inc.

McDonald, G. (2016). *Who really invented baseball?* Retrieved from https://www.seeker.com/who-really-invented-baseball-1771280977.html.

PBS. (2014). *African-American baseball.* Retrieved from http://www.pbs.org/opb/historydetectives/feature/african-american-baseball/.

Peterson, R. (1970). *Only the ball was white: A history of legendary black players and all-black professional teams.* Oxford: Oxford University Press.

Ruck, R. (2011). *Raceball: How the Major Leagues colonized the black and Latin game.* Boston: Beacon Press.

Thorn, J. (no date). *October 1845: The first recorded baseball games in New York.* Retrieved from https://sabr.org/gamesproj/game/october-1845-first-recorded-baseball-games-new-york.

Thorn, J. (2004). *Total baseball: The ultimate baseball encyclopedia.* Wilmington: Sport Media Pub.

Twain, M. (1889). TwainQuotes.com. Retrieved from http://www.twainquotes.com/Baseball.html.

Tygiel, J. (1983). *Baseball's great experiment: Jackie Robinson and his legacy.* Oxford: Oxford University Press.

Vaught, D. (2013). *The Farmers' game: Baseball in rural America.* Baltimore: Johns Hopkins University Press.

White, S. (1907). *Sol White's history of colored baseball with other documents on the early black game, 1886–1936.* Omaha: University of Nebraska Press.

Wilkerson, I. (2016). The long-lasting legacy of the Great Migration. Retrieved from https://www.smithsonianmag.com/history/long-lasting-legacy-great-migration-180960118/.

Wright, M. D. (2000). *The National Association of Base Ball Players, 1857–1870.* Jefferson: McFarland & Company.

Chapter 2
A Mini-history of Latin America and Professional Baseball

2.1 Background

It is beyond the scope of this book to detail the history of all countries where Latin American Major League Baseball players in the current study cohort were born. Briefly, these countries included Cuba, the Dominican Republic, Venezuela, Puerto Rico, Mexico and Panama. (Puerto Rico is a US territory, although for study purposes, it will be labeled a "country.") In addition, a very limited number of players in the study cohort were born in Nicaragua and Colombia. These 8 countries will be referred to in this book as the "Hispanic cohort countries."

The countries of Latin America are diverse, and the cohort countries reflect this. Nevertheless, the cohort countries share common historical threads. As was the case in the US, all the Hispanic cohort countries were conquered and colonized by European powers beginning in the fifteenth century. While the US was colonized by the British, the Hispanic cohort countries were colonized by the Spaniards.

The conquered territories were initially inhabited by indigenous populations who had virtually no previous contact with Europeans. Lacking immunity for common diseases experienced in Europe, up to 90% of indigenous populations in Latin America died due to epidemics of smallpox, typhus, influenza, measles and several other diseases (Montenegro and Stephens 2006). To meet cheap laborer needs resulting from widespread deaths among indigenous people, the European colonizers began importing slaves from Africa. The production of crops, such as sugar, tobacco, coffee and cotton, mainly on plantations that utilized slave labor, became the foundation of many Latin American economies. The Atlantic slave trade continued for more than 350 years (Gilder Lehrman Institute of American History no date).

While slavery had developed in Africa prior to the start of the slave trade, it was more like European serfdom and not nearly as malevolent as the form of slavery that subsequently emerged in the US (Davidson 1988). Moreover, while Africans living in Spanish colonized countries were considered property, they were sometimes charged with responsibilities that enabled them to function as intermediaries between Europeans and indigenous people. A limited number of African slaves in Latin American countries were able to buy their way out of bondage (Pino 1997).

Trading African slaves and their use as laborers proved to be an economically profitable business and by 1870, 7 mainly European countries had shipped about 12.5 million Africans to North America, Latin America and the Caribbean, although about 2 million of these individuals died in route to their targeted locations (Gates Jr. 2014).

By the late seventeenth and early eighteenth centuries, pressure mounted on Spain and other European countries to end the slave trade, and eventually, to free the slaves. With strong abolitionist and diplomatic efforts, as well as the emergence of slave revolts throughout the New World, the legal end of slavery came to most Latin American countries in the mid-1800s. The US in 1865, Cuba in 1886, and Brazil in 1888 were the last countries in the New World to abolish slavery (Encyclopedia.com 2006). Moreover, as was the case in the US, the legal abolition of slavery did not result in the end of racism, discrimination and inequalities that disadvantaged Afro-Latinos (Andrews 2018).

Social and sexual relations between Europeans, indigenous people, and Africans in Latin America were common and resulted in racially and ethnically blended offspring. The Spanish conquerors as well as the Church sought biological and cultural purity, but the mixing of the different populations made this difficult. In fact, the Spaniards implemented elaborate systems to track the race and ethnicity of Latin American inhabitants by attempting to monitor the genealogy of every person (Martinez 2008). However, in addition to incomplete and inconsistent records, each successive generation resulted in more complicated combinations of intermixed people, and eventually, racial classification systems were abandoned.

The legal abolition of slavery in Latin America was deceptive since it failed to provide social, political or economic equality for Afro-descendants, and the racial and class inequalities linked to the slave economies persisted. In territories subjugated by Spain, the conquerors occupied the top realm in a social pyramid that pushed many Blacks and indigenous people to the bottom. The pyramid's middle level was tied to "…ancestry, appearance… occupation and wealth" (Wade 2008). Compared to those occupying the top and bottom rungs of this class system, placement in the middle was ambiguous and contentious in Latin America.

2.2 Race/Ethnicity and Discrimination in Latin America Versus the US

While race in the US developed into a white and African-American dichotomy, Latin America evolved as "a continuum of color" (Eakin 2007). Because race was more complex and nuanced in Latin America relative to the US, there was more fluidity with respect to race and social class. And when race was used as justification to discriminate, it was not always clear who would be affected, particularly among individuals in the middle part of the Latin American stratification system. "If there is little agreement on who is black (or white or indigenous), how can discrimination take place in any systematic way? In contrast, in the US, there was generally a clearer definition of racial identity, based on a few key categories: black, white, Native American …" (Wade 2008).

The stratification system that would continue in many Latin American countries following the end of formal slavery placed Afro-Latinos and indigenous people, and to a lesser extent, mixed-race individuals, in economically, socially, and politically disadvantaged situations. The absence of educational opportunities, widespread poverty, and underrepresentation in government did little to help those who found themselves at or near the bottom of the stratification system.

2.3   Hispanics in Baseball

The following is a brief description of how baseball evolved in 6 of the Hispanic cohort countries, with a special focus on Cuba, the first Latin American country where baseball developed and grew.

2.3.1   Cuba

Sent to the US for a good college education, the Guillo brothers are credited with bringing baseball to their native country, Cuba, in 1864, and within a decade, the sport became enormously popular there. While the game began as a rich man's sport in the US, baseball had mass appeal in Cuba owing to its simplicity and low cost. Around 1880, an amateur Cuban league was created that eventually became the Cuban Winter League. Not so coincidentally, the first Cuban professional League emerged only 2 years after the National League of Major League Baseball was formed. This professional baseball league operated continuously until the rise of Fidel Castro in the late 1950s.

Enthusiasm over the game of baseball in Cuba during the latter part of the nineteenth century coincided with its struggle for independence and modernization. Choosing baseball over bullfighting was analogous to choosing independence over Spanish domination and became part of Cuba's "rehearsal for democracy" (Perez 1994).

The earlier Cuban professional baseball teams excluded blacks, but by the beginning of the twentieth century, professional baseball in Cuba became integrated. Cuban baseball teams, comprised of multiracial players, barnstormed and created their own leagues in the US around the beginning of the twentieth century. One team, the Cuban Stars, played so well that they were granted charter membership in the US Negro National League in 1920. In contrast to dark-skinned Afro-Cubans, several Spanish ancestry Cubans with light skin color played in Minor League organizations within Major League Baseball as early as the beginning of the twentieth century (Eschevarria no date).

In the aftermath of political turmoil in Cuba that resulted in Civil War, the US occupied the country between 1906 and 1909. This greatly increased Cuban exposure to US baseball with both Negro League and Major League Baseball teams scheduling exhibition games on the island. In 1911, the first 2 Cuban players were signed to Major League Baseball contracts. While the lighter-skin signees would pass as whites to many, there were other, more talented dark-skinned Hispanic players who failed to get contracts. The "Gentleman's Agreement" that banned African-Americans from baseball for the first half of the twentieth century applied to anyone with black skin (Negro League Baseball Museum 2006) including many Afro-Latinos. Negro League players especially enjoyed playing baseball in Cuba. While far from an ideal country when it came to race, Cuba emerged as a model for multiracial, international baseball play at the highest levels. "The [Cuban Baseball League] was an anomaly, the only place in the world where the best professional ballplayers of all nations and colors competed with and against each other" (Ruck 2011).

2.3.2 Venezuela

Baseball spread to Venezuela during the last decade of the nineteenth century. As was the case in Cuba, it was a group of young men attending US universities who introduced the game to the country. Initially, players were from high-class social clubs in Caracas, but later the game was more broadly adopted. The sport rapidly gained popularity throughout Venezuela and the country's first baseball stadium was built within a few years. Interestingly, the first organized baseball game in Venezuela was billed as a "new kind of Chess game" (Baseball Reference 2013). By 1920, there were 30 organized baseball teams who played in 10 different ballparks in the city of Maracaibo alone (Baseball Reference 2013). When oil was discovered in Venezuela in 1922, money flowed into the country attracting white and Negro League players from the US to play baseball. By 1927, professional baseball began in Venezuela and in 1945, a professional baseball Winter League was formed. Since 1939, more than 350 baseball players from Venezuela have played in the Major Leagues.

2.3.3 Mexico

An early form of baseball may go back to the mid-nineteenth century in Mexico when the game was introduced by US military personnel involved in the Mexican-American War. The game spread throughout the country when US soldiers helped lay tracks for a new train system known as the Monterrey-Tampico railway (Hughson 2018). During the latter part of the 1800s, employees of American companies doing business in Mexico helped spread the game throughout the country. Professional baseball in Mexico was first played in 1925. A triple-A Minor League system (the highest level possible) known as the Mexican League, began in 1967 and continues today. Despite intense competition from soccer, baseball persists as a very popular sport in Mexico and contributes dozens of players to Major League Baseball.

2.3.4 Puerto Rico

The influence of Cubans and Americans was integral to bringing baseball to Puerto Rico. Because of the Spanish-American War, there were large numbers of American military personnel stationed in Puerto Rico who helped expose and popularize the game. Following the War, a treaty with Spain, would make Puerto Rico a US possession. By 1918, Negro League teams as well as teams comprised of Cuban All-Stars played exhibition games in Puerto Rico. Winter league baseball in Puerto Rico, which began in 1940, continues today. Since the debut of Hiram Bithorn, a Puerto-Rican-born pitcher with the Chicago Cubs in 1942, more than 260 players from the island have played Major League Baseball. In fact, some of the greatest Major League Baseball players of all-time like Roberto Clemente, Orlando Cepeda, Roberto Alomar, and Iván Rodríguez, all Hall of Famers, were born in Puerto Rico.

2.3.5 Dominican Republic

The Dominican Republic is another Latin American country in which Cuba played a pivotal role in introducing baseball. In part, this was due to the Ten Years War (1868–1878), an integral part of Cuba's fight for independence from Spain. When large numbers of Cubans fled the war to the Dominican Republic, they brought with them their love of baseball. By the early 1920s, a professional league comprised of 4 teams formed the Dominican League. A military coup in 1930 led by Rafael Trujillo resulted in the demise of professional baseball in the Dominican Republic around 1937 (MLB.com/DR 2018). Nevertheless, amateur baseball flourished and by 1951 the Winter League of the Dominican Republic was reestablished. Currently, there are more Major League Baseball players born in the Dominican Republic than from any other Latin American country (Wikipedia 2018).

2.3.6 Panama

Baseball was played in Panama during the 1880s when the country was a province of Colombia. Upon procuring its independence in 1903, Panama signed a treaty with the US to build a canal beginning the following year. The work on the canal increased Panamanian exposure to baseball particularly among West Indian workers who participated in the construction effort. Not until 1945 was the Professional Base-ball League of Panama established. Although this organization existed continuously through 1972, it subsequently folded due to economic issues, replaced by a strong amateur baseball presence (Reid 2010).

2.4   Journeys Travelled by Hispanic Players to Major League Baseball

The journeys travelled by Latin American players to Major League Baseball vary a great deal but have often been marred by personal difficulty and danger. More than a few individuals, including several Hispanic players in the study cohort have risked their lives to play Major League Baseball (Weeks 2017). Many Latin Americans players have emerged from impoverished conditions with little or no education to make it to baseball's pinnacle. Once they arrive in the US, they can be challenged by cultural differences like dietary changes and language barriers. Being born in Latin America and playing in baseball's Major League is a tremendous personal and professional accomplishment that often comes with financial rewards that can have life-changing consequences.

References

Andrews, G. R. (2018). Inequality: Race, class, gender. In A. de la Fuente & G. R. Andrews (Eds.), *Afro-Latin American studies*. UK: Cambridge University Press.

Baseball Reference (2013). *History of baseball in Venezuela*. Retrieved from https://www.baseball-reference.com/bullpen/History_of_baseball_in_Venezuela.

Davidson, B. (1988). *The African slave trade*. Boston: Little Brown and Company.

Eakin, M. C. (2007). *The history of Latin America: Collision of cultures*. New York: St. Martin's Griffin.

Encyclopedia.com (2006). *Emancipation in Latin America and the Caribbean. Encyclopedia of African-American culture and history*. Retrieved from https://www.encyclopedia.com/history/encyclopedias-almanacs-transcripts-and-maps/emancipation-latin-america-and-caribbean.

Eschevarria, R. G. (no date). Latin Americans in Major League Baseball through the first years of the 21st century. *Encyclopedia Britannica*. Retrieved from https://www.britannica.com/topic/Latin-Americans-in-Major-League-Baseball-910675.

Gates Jr., H. L. (2014). *How many slaves landed in the US?* Retrieved from https://www.theroot.com/how-many-slaves-landed-in-the-us-1790873989.

Gilder Lehrman Institute of American History (no date). H*istorical context: Facts about the slave trade and slavery*. Retrieved from https://www.gilderlehrman.org/content/historical-context-facts-about-slave-trade-and-slavery.

Hughson, C. (2018). *Baseball in Mexico*. Retrieved from http://mopupduty.com/baseball-in-mexico-040618/.

Martinez, M. E. (2008). *Genealogical fictions*. Stanford: Stanford University Press.

MLB.com/DR (2018). *History*. Retrieved from http://mlb.mlb.com/dr/history.jsp.

Montenegro, R. A., & Stephens, C. (2006). Indigenous health in Latin America and the Caribbean. *The Lancet, 367*(9525), 1850–1869.

Negro League Baseball Museum, eMuseum Glossary (2006) Retrieved from http://coe.k-state.edu/annex/nlbemuseum/glossary.html.

Perez, L. A. (1994). Between baseball and bullfighting: The quest for nationality in Cuba, 1868–1898. *Journal of American History, 81*(2), 493–517.

Pino, J. C. (1997). *Teaching the history of race in Latin America. Perspectives on history.* Retrieved from https://www.historians.org/publications-and-directories/perspectives-on-history/october-1997/teaching-the-history-of-race-in-latin-america.

Reid, L. M. (2010). *Baseball's roots in Panama.* Retrieved from https://thesilverpeopleheritage.wordpress.com/2010/01/31/baseballs-roots-in-panama/.

Ruck, R. (2011). *Raceball: How the Major Leagues colonized the Black and Latin game.* Boston: Beacon Press.

Wade, P. (2008). *Race in Latin America.* In D. Poole (Ed.), *A companion to Latin American anthropology,* Chapter 9. Oxford: Blackwell Publishing Ltd.

Weeks, J. (2017). *Latino stars in Major League Baseball.* Lanham: Rowman and Littlefield.

Wikipedia (2018). List *of current Major League Baseball players by nationality.* Retrieved from https://en.wikipedia.org/wiki/List_of_current_Major_League_Baseball_players_by_nationality.

Chapter 3
Literature and Statistical Review of Race/Hispanic Origin and Mortality

3.1 General Population Mortality Statistics

Prior chapters have provided context with respect to race/Hispanic origin and the evolution of baseball in the US, as well as the Hispanic cohort countries. Now, the focus turns to the primary topic of this book, mortality. Before moving on to the empirical analyses of mortality and race/Hispanic origin among individuals who played Major League Baseball, it is helpful to review the literature and interpret existing statistics related to mortality among the 3 groups of interest in the current study.

This chapter is divided into 2 parts addressing mortality as it relates to race and Hispanic origin. The first part of the review focuses on mortality gathered from general population statistics, while the second part examines the mortality literature among professional athletes. The US general population review is derived from vital statistics data, i.e., death certificates, published by the Centers for Disease Control and Prevention (CDC) of the National Center of Health Statistics (2018), hereafter called the "CDC data." The importance and significance of death certificates from a public health and public policy perspective cannot be emphasized enough. "At both the state and national level, mortality data compiled from death certificates is used to track disease trends, set public health policies, and allocate health and research funding" (Brooks and Reed 2015).

There are, however, limitations associated with the use of death certificates. This includes cause of death and ethnicity classification errors. Cause of death errors do not apply to the current study since all-cause mortality is the focus. Ethnicity misclassification has been dropping over time and is currently estimated to be a problem for about 3% of Hispanics (Arias et al. 2016). According to the CDC: "Race and ethnicity reporting on the death certificate continues to be excellent for the white and black populations [and]… is reasonably good for… Hispanic[s]" (National Center of Health Statistics 2018).

© The Author(s), under exclusive license to Springer Nature Switzerland AG 2019
J. S. Markowitz, *Mortality Among Hispanic and African-American Players After Desegregation in Major League Baseball*, SpringerBriefs in Public Health, https://doi.org/10.1007/978-3-030-17280-0_3

In their reporting of vital statistics, the CDC uses terms like 'Black or African-Americans" and "Hispanic or Latino." Hence, these same terms will be used whenever the CDC race/Hispanic origin data is cited in the text or table displays in this chapter. Because the current study pertains to male baseball players, the general population literature review will address men only.

Together, these 2 mortality-related literature reviews, i.e., general population and professional athletes, should help frame the key study hypotheses that will be specified in Chap. 4.

3.2 CDC General Population Mortality-Related Statistics

The review of CDC general population vital statistics includes life expectancy at birth, all-cause death rates and death rates for the 2 most common causes of death in the US, i.e., heart disease and cancer. To show trends over time, statistics are reported for selected years between 1970 and 2014. Prior to 2006, life expectancy statistics for whites and African-Americans included persons of Hispanic and non-Hispanic origin. Beginning in 2006, life expectancy statistics are reported separately for "Whites, not Hispanics," "Blacks, not Hispanics" as well as "Hispanics." Death rate data for "Black or African-Americans" includes Hispanics and non-Hispanics. Beginning in 1990, death rate data are reported for "Whites, not Hispanic or Latino."

3.3 Life Expectancy

Life expectancy at birth is an estimate of the number of years that an individual or group can expect to live at the time of their birth. This estimate is based on age-specific death rates that are available for each year of birth. According to the CDC "Differences in life expectancy among various demographic subpopulations, including racial and ethnic groups, may reflect subpopulation differences in a range of factors such as socioeconomic status, access to medical care, and the prevalence of specific risk factors in a particular subpopulation" (National Center for Health Statistics 2016).

See Table 3.1 for a summary of US general population life expectancy statistics for males for selected years between 1970 and 2014 (National Center for Health Statistics 2016). Life expectancy at birth in 1970 is 68 years for male whites and 60 years for male "Blacks or African-Americans." By 1980, life expectancy for whites increases to 70.7 years and continues to increase through 2000 to 74.7 years. Life expectancy for Blacks or African-Americans also increases over time to 68.2 years in the year 2000. The between-race gap in life expectancy favoring whites by about 6–8 years fails to change much between 1970 and 2000. Beginning in 2006, the between-race

Table 3.1 Life expectancy at birth (in years) for US males between 1970 and 2014 by race/Hispanic origin

Race/Hispanic origin	Year						
	1970	1980	1990	2000	2006	2010	2014
Life expectancy							
White[a]	68.0	70.7	72.7	74.7	See row below		
White, not Hispanic	Not available	Not available	Not available	Not available	75.7	76.4	76.5
Black or African-American[a]	60.0	63.8	64.5	68.2	See row below		
Black, not Hispanic	Not available	Not available	Not available	Not available	69.5	71.4	72
Hispanic	Not available	Not available	Not available	Not available	77.5	78.5	79.2

Source National Center for Health Statistics Health, United States, 2017, Hyattsville, Maryland, 2018, US Government Printing Office, Washington, D.C., Table 15. Located at https://www.cdc.gov/nchs/data/hus/hus15.pdf
[a]Includes persons of Hispanic and non-Hispanic origin

mortality difference decline to 6.2 years, and then further narrow in 2010 to 5 years. By 2014, the between-race difference among US males is at its lowest recorded point of 4.5 years (National Center for Health Statistics 2016).

The first publication of life expectancy statistics for Hispanics by the CDC was in 2006. Between 2006 and 2014, life expectancy for Hispanics, relative to non-Hispanic whites, is about 2–3 years older and, relative to Blacks or African-Americans, about 7 years older.

3.4 All-Cause Death Rates

Table 3.2 summarizes age-adjusted, all-cause, heart disease and malignant neoplasm mortality rates per 100,000 US general population for male residents for selected years between 1970 and 2014 based on race and Hispanic origin. In 1970, Black or African-American males have an all-cause death rate of 1873.9 per 100,000 residents which is higher than the rates for whites who average 1513.7. In 1990, all-cause death rate data for Hispanics or Latinos are reported for the first time and their rate of 886.4 is far lower than Whites, not Hispanic or Latinos (1170.9) and Black or African-Americans who average 1644.5. By 2014, all-cause death rates drop substantially for all 3 groups with rates of 626.8 for Hispanics or Latinos, 872.3 for Whites, not Hispanic or Latinos and 1034 for Blacks or African-Americans.

Table 3.2 Age-adjusted all-cause, heart disease and malignant neoplasm death rates per 100,000 US resident population for selected years between 1970 and 2014 by race/Hispanic origin (males)

Race/Hispanic origin	Year				
	1970	1980	1990	2000	2014
All-cause death rates					
White[a]	1513.7	1317.6	1165.9	1029.4	853.4
White, not Hispanic or Latino	Not available	Not available	1170.9	1317.6	853.4
Black or African-American[a]	1873.9	1697.8	1644.5	1403.5	1034.0
Hispanic or Latino	Not available	Not available	886.4	818.1	626.8
Heart disease death rates					
White[a]	640.2	539.6	409.2	316.7	210.0
White, not Hispanic or Latino	Not available	Not available	413.6	319.9	215.2
Black or African-American[a]	607.3	561.4	485.4	392.5	259.5
Hispanic or Latino	Not available	Not available	270.0	238.2	145.7
Malignant neoplasms death rates					
White[a]	244.8	265.1	272.2	243.9	193.0
White, not Hispanic or Latino	Not available	Not available	276.7	247.7	197.7
Black or African-American[a]	227.6	291.9	397.9	340.3	231.9
Hispanic or Latino	Not available	Not available	174.7	171.7	135.9

Source National Center for Health Statistics Health, United States, 2017, Hyattsville, Maryland, 2018, US Government Printing Office, Washington, D.C., Tables 21, 22 and 24 Located at https://www.cdc.gov/nchs/hus/contents2015.htm#017
[a]Includes persons of Hispanic and non-Hispanic origin

3.5   Heart Disease and Cancer Death Rates

Heart disease and cancer consistently represent the top 2 leading causes of death in the US general population. In 2015, about 46–47% of all male deaths in the US are attributable to 1 of these 2 causes with just slight differences in the rates between the 2 diseases. No other cause of death among males in the US general population encompasses more than 7% of all deaths in 2015 (CDC 2018).

Male death rate data for heart disease and cancer, the latter referred to as "malignant neoplasms" by the CDC, for selected years between 1970 and 2014 broken down by race and Hispanic origin are displayed in Table 3.2. The trends reflected in this table are very similar to the ones presented previously for overall death rates. With few exceptions, heart disease and malignant neoplasm death rates for all 3 groups decline over time with clear mortality disadvantages evident for Black or African-Americans. Relative to whites, African-American males have higher heart disease and malignant neoplasm death rates for the 4 timepoints shown in Table 3.2 beginning in 1980. In addition, Hispanics have the lowest heart disease and malignant neoplasm death rates of the 3 groups in 1990, 2000 and 2014; the 3 timepoints with data available for Hispanics (National Center for Health Statistics 2016).

Several conclusions can be drawn from the CDC general population life expectancy and death rate data. First, over time life expectancy has lengthened, and death rates have declined for all 3 groups of interest. Second, during the limited period that CDC data have been available for Hispanics, life expectancy is longer and death rates are lower compared to African-Americans as well as non-Hispanic whites. Finally, life expectancy and death rates are more similar between Hispanics and non-Hispanic whites than they are between African-Americans and non-Hispanic whites.

3.6 The Hispanic Paradox

Despite being at the low end on educational attainment and income spectrums, available CDC statistics consistently document superior mortality outcomes among Hispanics living in the US relative to other groups including non-Hispanic whites. This so-called "Hispanic Paradox" has been chronicled in numerous studies since 1980 (Franzini et al. 2001; Ruiz et al. 2013; Markides and Coreil 1986).

One of the earliest journal articles documenting what appeared to be an epidemiological mortality paradox for Hispanics relative to whites was published in 1986 by Markides and Coreil (1986). These authors found *similarities* between Hispanics living in the Southwest US, mainly Mexican-Americans, and non-Hispanic whites on infant mortality, life expectancy, and mortality rates for certain cancers as well as cardiovascular disease. Beginning in the 1990s, additional research was conducted to examine this further and the concept of a Hispanic Paradox evolved. In fact, several of the subsequent studies document outright mortality advantages, rather than similarities, for selected Hispanic populations relative to non-Hispanic whites (Markides et al. 1997; Sorlie et al. 1993). "The evidence in support of the [Hispanic mortality] advantage has been based on a variety of data sources, including vital statistics, community surveys linked to National Death Index data, Medicare data linked to application records for Social Security cards maintained [by] the Social Security Administration …., and mortality follow-ups by individual regional studies" (Markides and Eschbach 2005).

In several studies, the Hispanic Paradox is shown to be evident primarily within older age groups (Markides et al. 1997; Hummer et al. 2004). It has also been determined that the paradox is most apparent in immigrant Hispanics (Hummer et al. 2000), especially Mexican immigrants (Palloni and Arias 2004). The paradox is not, however, readily evident among US-born Hispanics (Singh and Hiatt 2006).

Nevertheless, questions have been raised regarding the Hispanic Paradox. The paradox seems more difficult to establish in research where all deaths within a population have been identified (Smith and Bradshaw 2006). Other potential issues with the Hispanic Paradox have included "...data problems such as a lack of comparability in reporting of Hispanic origin in vital statistics and census records, age misreporting, and difficulties in linking persons of Hispanic origin among various data sources..." (Turra and Elo 2008).

Feasible alternative hypotheses have been proposed attempting to explain the apparent mortality advantage of Hispanics living in the US. One explanation that has received considerable attention in the scientific literature is the "unhealthy out-migrant hypothesis" (Pablos-Mendez 1994), commonly referred to as the "salmon bias." Briefly, this hypothesis postulates that out-migration may be more frequent among US residents born in Latin American countries after their health deteriorates. Such people could return to their native countries for cultural and other reasons, particularly at older ages, and die in their home countries rather than in the US. As a result, US death certificates are not issued for these individuals, and they fail to be counted in US mortality statistics. To the extent that this occurs, this has the effect of underestimating US death rates and overestimating life expectancy among Hispanics who continue to reside in the US. If the salmon bias is a realistic explanation for the Hispanic Paradox, it would logically have its greatest impact among older individuals, possibly in failing health, as well as immigrants from countries more proximate to the US, like Mexico. In fact, these are 2 of the groups, whose mortality outcomes provide the strongest evidence for the paradox (Markides and Eschbach 2005).

In brief, while there has been substantial support for the Hispanic Paradox from a variety of sources in the scientific literature, questions exist, and alternative hypotheses cannot be readily ruled-out. Special groups, like former Major League Baseball players have not been studied in relationship to the Hispanic Paradox or the salmon bias. The current study contains too few Hispanics to confidently address questions related to the paradox. Moreover, this study is focused on a very special group of Hispanics, namely former professional baseball players, and their mortality experiences could be dissimilar to their counterparts in the general population. Nevertheless, by studying former Major League Baseball players born in Latin American countries, clues can be provided that might help guide future research efforts related to the study of the Hispanic Paradox.

3.7 Professional Athlete Literature

Baseball, basketball and football players have contributed to our understanding of mortality risk among professional athletes based on race, but there is little or no information on this topic as it relates to individuals of Hispanic origin.

3.7.1 Baseball

Several published studies have examined mortality among former Major League Baseball players (Panjer 1993; Saint Onge et al. 2008; Reynolds and Day 2012). However, comparisons of mortality outcomes based on race, and especially Hispanic origin, are quite limited. Life expectancy was investigated by Saint Onge and colleagues (2008) in their study of 6772 Major League Baseball players who debuted between 1902 and 2004. However, undisclosed data limitations did not allow for life expectancy comparisons based on race/ethnicity.

3.7.2 Basketball

Critical literature on mortality and race among professional basketball players comes from 2 publications (Lawler et al. 2012; Markowitz 2018). However, neither of these studies could reasonably examine mortality among Hispanic basketball players. While the number of NBA players born in Latin American countries has increased over time, there are too few Hispanic players to study in a meaningful way.

Lawler and colleagues (2012) conducted a 59-year historical cohort study of more than 3300 professional basketball players who played in the US anytime between 1946 and 2005. In all 4 Cox regressions conducted with slightly different sets of variables, there is about a 70–85% increased risk of mortality among African-Americans compared to whites that, in all cases, is statistically significant.

Markowitz (2018) compared mortality risk between African-American and white NBA players who played in the League between 1960 and 1986 using multivariate Cox models that control for year of birth, BMI, years of career playing experience, and birthplace region. The results indicate that African-Americans have a statistically significant (86%) increased mortality risk relative to whites. When only significant variables are retained in a second Cox analysis, the mortality risk for African-Americans remains elevated by 58% and continues to be significant (Markowitz 2018).

3.7.3 Football

In 1994, researchers from the National Institute for Occupational Safety and Health (NIOSH) reported on the causes, risks and rates of mortality among about 6800 former NFL players who were active between 1959 and 1988 (Baron and Rinsky 1994). The study uses a vital status end date of December 31, 1991 and because of this, the median age of the study cohort is only about 41 years. Predictably, the number of reported deaths, 103 or about 2% of the cohort, is low. Nevertheless, comparisons of mortality to the general population reveal a decreased risk of dying among the NFL players relative to the general population. Despite this advantage for the entire

NIOSH cohort, linemen have elevated rates of cardiovascular mortality compared to the general population. As a follow-up to this finding, within-player analyses are conducted to identify risk factors for cardiovascular deaths. In "internal analyses," which divide the cohort into whites and non-whites, there is a 70% significant increased risk of cardiovascular mortality for non-whites in analyses that separately control for BMI and player position (Baron and Rinsky 1994).

The NIOSH researchers later conducted a 17-year follow-up study with a subgroup of their 1994 cohort limited to players who had at least 5 years of pension-credited service in the NFL (Baron et al. 2012). Internal risk factor analyses of cardiovascular mortality risk examine the effect of BMI, era of play, player position and race. When race is entered in 3 of the 4 Cox regressions, hazard ratios predicting cardiovascular mortality risk ranges from 1.57 to 1.71 for non-whites, and in all 3 instances, is statistically significant (Baron et al. 2012).

Markowitz (2018) studied all-cause mortality risk factors among former NFL players who played in the league anytime between 1960 and 1986. Just over 6500 US-born players have non-missing race data and are included in the analyses of race. In a Cox regression that control for year of birth, African-American NFL players have a 59% increased risk of dying compared to white players. In multivariate analyses that control for year of birth plus all other significant predictors of all-cause mortality, African-American race is a significant independent risk factor for mortality with a hazard ratio that reflects a 30% increased risk of dying relative to whites (Markowitz 2018).

Attention will now be turned to the empirical study of former Major League Baseball players that is the focus of this book. The first step will be to delineate the methods and specify the hypotheses. This will be followed by preliminary statistical analyses, and then increasingly more sophisticated analyses that consider other potentially important variables.

References

Arias, E., Heron, M., & Hakes, J. K. (2016). The validity of race and Hispanic-origin reporting on death certificates in the United States: An update. *Vital and Health Statistics, Series, 2, 172(172)*, 1–23.

Baron, S. L., & Rinsky, R. (1994). *Health hazard evaluation report, National Football League players mortality study*. Report No. HETA 88-085. Atlanta: Centers for Disease Control and Prevention/National Institute for Occupational Safety and Health. Retrieved from https://www.cdc.gov/niosh/hhe/reports/pdfs/1988-0085-letter.pdf?id=10.26616/NIOSHHETA88085.

Baron, S. L., Hein, M. J., Lehman, E., & Gersic, C. M. (2012). Body mass index, playing position, race, and the cardiovascular mortality of retired professional football players. *American Journal of Cardiology, 109*, 889–896.

Brooks, E. G., & Reed, K. D. (2015). Principles and pitfalls: A guide to death certification. *Clinical Medicine and Research, 13*(2), 74–82.

CDC (2018). *Leading causes of death in males, 2015*. Retrieved from https://www.cdc.gov/healthequity/lcod/men/2015/race-ethnicity/index.htm.

Franzini, L., Ribble, J. C., & Keddie, A. M. (2001). Understanding the Hispanic paradox. *Ethnicity and Disease, 11,* 496–518.

Hummer, R. A., Rogers, R. G., Amir, S. H., Forbes, D., & Frisbie, W. P. (2000). Adult mortality differentials among Hispanic subgroups and non-Hispanic Whites. *Social Science Quarterly, 81,* 459–476.

Hummer, R. A., Benjamins, M. R., & Rogers, R. G. (2004). Racial and ethnic disparities in health and mortality among the U.S. elderly population. In R. A. Bulatao & N. B. Anderson (Eds.), *Understanding racial and ethnic differences in health in late life: A research agenda.* Washington: National Academy Press.

Lawler, T., Lawler, F., Gibson, J., & Murray, R. (2012). Does the African-American-white mortality gap persist after playing professional basketball? A 50-year historical cohort study. *Annals of Epidemiology, 22,* 406–412.

Markides, K. S., & Coreil, J. (1986). The health of Southwestern Hispanics: An epidemiologic paradox. *Public Health Reports, 101,* 253–265.

Markides, K. S., & Eschbach, K. (2005). Aging, migration, and mortality: Current status of research on the Hispanic Paradox. *The Journals of Gerontology, Series B, 60*(2), 68–75.

Markides, K. S., Rudkin, L., Angel, R. J., & Espino, D. V. (1997). Health status of Hispanic elderly in the United States. In L. G. Martin & B. Soldo (Eds.), *Racial and ethnic differences in the health of older Americans.* Washington: National Academy Press.

Markowitz, J. S. (2018). *Mortality and its risk factors among professional athletes: A comparison between former NBA and NFL players.* Cham: Springer.

National Center for Health Statistics. (2016). *Health, United States, 2015: With special feature on racial and ethnic health disparities.* Washington, D.C.: US Government Printing Office.

Pablos-Mendez, A. (1994). Mortality among Hispanics. *JAMA, 271*(16), 1237. (letter; comment on: JAMA, 1993, 270(20), 2464–2468).

Palloni, A., & Arias, E. (2004). Paradox lost: Explaining the Hispanic adult mortality advantage. *Demography, 4,* 385–415.

Panjer, H. H. (1993). Mortality differences by handedness: Survival analysis for a right-truncated sample of baseball players. *Transactions of Society of Actuaries, 45,* 257–274.

Reynolds, R. & Day, S. (2012). Life expectancy and comparative mortality of Major League Baseball players, 1900–1999. *WebmedCentral Sports Medicine, 3*(5). Retrieved from http://www.webmedcentral.com/article_view/3380.

Ruiz, J. M., Steffen, P., & Smith, Y. B. (2013). Hispanic mortality paradox: A systematic review and meta-analysis of the longitudinal literature. *American Journal of Public Health.* Retrieved from https://ajph.aphapublications.org/doi/abs/10.2105/AJPH.2012.301103.

Saint Onge, J. M., Rogers, R. G., & Krueger, P. M. (2008). MLB players' life expectancies. *Social Science Quarterly, 89*(3), 817–830.

Singh, G. K., & Hiatt, R. A. (2006). Trends and disparities in socioeconomic and behavioural characteristics, life expectancy, and cause-specific mortality of native-born and foreign-born populations in the United States, 1979–2003. *International Journal of Epidemiology, 35*(4), 903–919.

Smith, D. P., & Bradshaw, B. S. (2006). Rethinking the Hispanic Paradox: Death rates and life expectancy for US non-Hispanic white and Hispanic populations. *American Journal of Public Health, 96*(9), 1686–1692.

Sorlie, P. D., Backlund, M. S., Johnson, J. K., & Rogat, F. (1993). Mortality by Hispanic status in the United States. *JAMA, 270,* 2646–2648.

Turra, C. M., & Elo, I. T. (2008). The impact of Salmon Bias on the Hispanic mortality advantage. *Population Research and Policy Review, 27,* 515–530.

Part II
Empirical Study Description and Preliminary Results

Chapter 4
Study Methods

4.1 Study Objective and Design

This is a retrospective cohort study based on player-specific and baseball-related data. The primary objective of this study is to determine whether there are differences in all-cause mortality risk among 3 groups of former Major League Baseball players, i.e., African-Americans, Hispanics, and non-Hispanic whites, who participated in the League during the 40 years following the end of segregation in baseball beginning in 1947. The study cohort includes all individuals who played Major League Baseball anytime between 1947 and 1986. These years were selected for several reasons. First, Major League Baseball's color barrier was broken in 1947. Not only did this open the door to a slow but steady influx of African-American players into Major League Baseball, but dark-skinned Hispanics, who previously had not been welcomed into the League, were then permitted to play as well (Stewart and Kennedy 2002). Only a small percentage of players who played Major League Baseball after 1986 will be deceased by the beginning of 2018. Given the costs and efforts to collect data on additional (younger) players, the large majority of whom are still alive, the decision was made to end data collection with individuals who played in 1986.

In retrospective database studies, it is sometimes difficult or impossible to obtain data on some variables of interest. In an ideal world, a mortality study would include variables likely to impact on illness and well-being, such as medical conditions, cigarette smoking, alcohol and drug use, exercise, nutrition, and family history. However, when the research is based on historical records that go back decades, the available variables may be limited. Although this is the case with respect to the current study, the variables considered in this book do allow for a reasonable test of the study hypotheses and should add significantly to existing knowledge in this area.

4.2   Data Sources

This study uses retrospective data from a variety of sources. The main data source is the Baseball Reference web-site (Sports Reference LLC 2018) which is one of the leading Internet sports statistics sites in the world. According to the Society for American Baseball Research, known as SABR, "[Baseball Reference.com is] easily the best source for precalculated historical statistics" (SABR a no date). In fact, Baseball Reference essentially offers a complete statistical history of every Major League Baseball team and all players.

Players in the study cohort were identified by creating a database with the names and birth dates of every individual on a Major League Baseball team between 1947 and 1986. This information was obtained from the Baseball Reference web-site by clicking on each team listed in the "Teams" section, then "Franchise History," and subsequently each season beginning with 1947 and continuing through 1986 (Sports Reference LLC 2018). This same procedure was repeated for each Major League Baseball team in existence between 1947 and 1986. A Statistical Analysis System (SAS) program (SAS 2018) was written to extract all unique players based on their first and last names as well as their dates of birth.

4.3   Hypotheses

Based on existing general population and professional athlete mortality literature, it is hypothesized that mortality risk will be significantly elevated among former African-American Major League Baseball players compared to Hispanic and non-Hispanic white players. No significant difference in mortality risk is predicted between Hispanic and non-Hispanic white players. These hypothesized relationships are expected to persist after controlling for year of birth and other potentially important variables. Existing scientific literature provides a strong justification for expecting African-Americans to be the most disadvantaged group when it comes to mortality (see Chap. 3). While Hispanics living in the US fare better mortality-wise than non-Hispanic whites in vital statistics, the general population literature is less consistent. Moreover, there are no mortality comparisons in the literature between Hispanics and non-Hispanic baseball players; accordingly, the null hypothesis is predicted between these groups.

4.4   The Primary Independent Variable: Race/Hispanic Origin

As the main independent variable for this study, race/Hispanic origin is comprised of 3 groups:

- non-Hispanic African-Americans (hereafter called African-Americans)
- Hispanics
- non-Hispanic whites.

Hispanic in this study is defined as individuals born in Latin American countries or Puerto Rico. Birthplace information, including country of birth, is publicly available on the "Players" pages of Baseball Reference (Sports Reference LLC 2018).

The race of American-born players was captured using a multistep approach. Unlike variables, such as players' weight, height and date of birth, race is generally not a publicly available variable. Therefore, race was obtained using a variety of sources, methods and techniques that include:

- the book titled "A hard road to glory: Baseball" (Ashe Jr. 1993)
- select historical baseball facts
- pictures mainly from baseball collector cards.

Prior to his death in 1993, Arthur Ashe Jr. the American tennis star, wrote a series of books on the Black athlete, including one specifically on baseball (Ashe Jr. 1993). In each of these books, Ashe Jr. includes extensive lists of African-American athletes. These lists, however, are not exhaustive and have to be supplemented with other methods and sources.

In Major League Baseball, many historical facts exist with respect to players' race. A well-referenced Wikipedia piece called "List of first black Major League Baseball players" identifies the first African-American players for each Major League Baseball team as well as their start dates in the League (Wikipedia 2018). For example, in 1959, the Boston Red Sox was the last Major League Baseball team to sign an African-American player. The Detroit Tigers fielded their first African-American in 1958 and the Philadelphia Phillies did so in 1957. It can be safely concluded that individuals on these teams who played prior to these respective seasons were either white or born in Latin American countries. Several players born outside of the US and Latin America were dropped and excluded from all statistical analyses. For purposes of this study, individuals born in a Latin American country would automatically be placed into the Hispanic group of players. Based on the respective years that the other Major League Baseball teams fielded their first African-American player, the same logic is used to identify the race of hundreds of additional players.

Several other race-related historical baseball facts further facilitated the identification of race for dozens of additional African-American and non-Hispanic white players. For example, there were several all-Black colleges, and players who attended these schools were all coded as African-American. In many cases, the historical facts serve to confirm race for individuals who have already been identified via the Ashe Jr. book and/or player photos (described below).

More so than any other professional sport, baseball is known for its long and storied tradition of collector cards. The first card goes back to the 1860s when they appeared in packs of cigarettes as a means of increasing sales. These rectangular cardboard cards later appeared in the twentieth century in packages accompanied by a piece of bubble gum and were manufactured by numerous companies. On the front of most of these cards is a photo of a Major League Baseball player. The likely race of most players can be determined from these collector cards, which now appear on Internet sites including eBay, Amazon, Wal-Mart, Target and dozens of other sports memorabilia sites. Finally, Googling the names of former Major League Baseball players can yield hundreds of images of the players of interest.

Because race is essentially a subjective construct, there is no guarantee that a player who appears to be white or African-American on a collector card or an Internet image, identifies himself as being that race. There is also the possibility that specific players come from mixed racial and ethnic backgrounds. The fact is that any player can be misclassified based on a photo alone. Although the multistep approach used to identify player race should minimize error, complete accuracy is uncertain. In this study, it can be assumed that every Hispanic player is classified correctly since this category is based solely on published country of birth.

4.5 The Primary Dependent Variable: Time to All-Cause Mortality

Using a vital status end-date of January 1, 2018, the main dependent variable for this study is time to all-cause mortality, or simply all-cause mortality. Cause-specific mortality data on former Major League Baseball players are not available to this author. All players who died on or before January 1, 2018 will be classified as dead, and all others will be considered alive. Some players classified "alive" for purpose of this study, have died sometime between January 2, 2018 and the writing of this book. This is a small limitation, but without a real-time means of capturing player deaths, no other options are available.

Vital status is a simple alive/dead variable that does not consider age at death for those who have died, or the age of players still alive. Admittedly crude, vital status begins to be meaningful when year of birth is simultaneously considered. Hence, analyses of vital status will be stratified by year of birth categories (to be detailed below).

Time to death, or age on the designated end-date for players still alive (January 1, 2018), is a so-called "time-to-event" variable that will be analyzed using Cox proportional hazards regressions, or Cox regressions or models (Cox and Oakes 1984). This survival procedure can be used with multiple independent variables and covariates and estimates the time it takes to experience a specific event. For purposes of the current study, time to death is the focus. Players who have died are considered "uncensored" observations, while those still alive on January 1, 2018 are "censored." Age at death is known with respect to uncensored players and is considered in the Cox models. What is known about censored players is that they have "survived" to the end-date without experiencing death. For purposes of the survival analyses contained in this book, the age of censored players on January 1, 2018 is the critical data piece. In Cox proportional hazards regressions, individuals who are censored contribute to the number of players who are at risk of dying based on their age on the vital status end-date (Allison 2010).

In addition to baseball demographic and player-related information, such as height, weight, years of play, player position and handedness, the "Players" pages of Baseball Reference also provide vital status data that, when applicable, includes date of death (Sports Reference LLC 2018). Data obtained from these sites have been used successfully in several prior mortality research studies of professional athletes (Lawler et al. 2012; Markowitz 2016; Markowitz 2018).

The mortality data published on the Baseball Reference Internet pages has been double-checked with vital status data available at other sites and in other databases. For example, the Lahman Baseball database (2017) contains comprehensive Major League Baseball player death information in its "Master File." This database has been characterized by SABR as "… basically a standard Baseball Encyclopedia in downloadable form" (SABR a no date).

As a test of the validity of the mortality data found on the "Players" pages of the Baseball Reference Internet-site, vital status was compared with the death data found in the Lahman database. At the time that this validity test was conducted, the Lahman database was updated through the end of 2016. The vital status of 100 randomly selected players in the study cohort who were still alive plus 100 randomly selected players who had passed away (through the end of 2016) according to Baseball Reference were compared with the data compiled by Lahman. In all 200 instances, the vital status of the players matches between these two databases. In addition, the dates of death match with respect to the players who have passed away. These results increase confidence, although do not ensure, that the mortality information contained at the Baseball Reference site is accurate and complete.

Former Major League Baseball players often remain in the media spotlight for years after retiring from baseball and it is common for their death information to be published on additional Internet and non-Internet sites. While there are many published sources of such material, these tend not to be systematic or complete. Nevertheless, death information on former Major League Baseball players can be found at numerous sports and celebrity Internet-sites as well as more general publications that include the Baseball Almanac (2018), Sporting News (2017), Tributes (2017), Find-a-Grave.com (2017), and the Los Angeles Times (2017). In addition to the validity checks detailed above utilizing the Lahman database, additional checks were done to compare death data found at the Baseball Reference site with other mortality information sources listed in this paragraph and, again, no discrepancies were found. These additional checks focused on players who died at relatively young or old ages, i.e., under 40 or over 90 years, since these may be the most prone to error.

4.6   The Primary Covariate: Year of Birth

Mortality and age are statistically linked. Beginning around the early teen years, the probability of dying increases with each successive year (Social Security Administration no date). Hence, age must be viewed as an essential covariate in mortality studies. In this study, year of birth will serve as the main covariate. While date of birth would be more accurate than birth year, analyzing year of birth provides more comprehensible interpretations of the data. Year of birth will be used in the analysis as both a categorical and continuous variable, depending on the analysis being conducted. Continuous year of birth will be slightly more accurate, but again, its categorical counterpart may improve interpretability. The specific year of birth categories to be used in this study are as follows:

- 1905–1914
- 1915–1924
- 1925–1934
- 1935–1944
- 1945–1954
- 1955–1966.

Two players in the study cohort were born in 1966.

4.7   Other Variables

In addition to race/Hispanic origin, (the main independent variable), year of birth, (the primary covariate), and all-cause mortality, (the primary dependent variable), several additional items will be analyzed in this book. This will include educational attainment, body mass index (BMI), US birthplace region, years of Major League Baseball playing experience, playing position and handedness. Conceptually, these are all independent variables that may add to the prediction of mortality risk above and beyond what is already explained by race/Hispanic origin. Alternatively, these other variables could help to clarify any relationship that is uncovered between race/Hispanic origin and all-cause mortality. Each of these other variables will now be described.

4.7.1   Educational Attainment

Two independent sources are used to measure educational attainment in this study as follows:

- Player pages of Baseball Reference (Sports Reference LLC 2018)
- College Playing spreadsheet of the Lahman Baseball Database (2017).

Baseball Reference (Sports Reference LLC 2018) provides the names of the high schools and colleges attended by each player but does not indicate the number of years completed or whether the respective players graduated. The Lahman Baseball Database (2017) gives the number of years of college attendance for the sub-group of players who attended college in their "College Playing" database. In the rare instances where there was a discrepancy between these two educational attainment data sources, individual SABR biographies (SABR b no date) were consulted, if available.

Based on these information sources, the following 5 categories of educational attainment have been created:

- little or no high school
- at least some high school, but no college
- some college, but unknown number of years completed
- 1–2 years of college completed
- 3 or more years of college completed.

These categories are essentially ordinal, rather than continuous, and will be treated as categorical items in the analysis.

4.7.2 Body Mass Index (BMI)

BMI is a measure of weight that is adjusted for height. Playing-time BMI during the last year of play in Major League Baseball will be used in this study. Height and weight data have beem obtained from the Players pages of Baseball Reference (Sports Reference LLC 2018).

According to the World Health Organization, (W.H.O. 2008), BMI can be aggregated into 4 categories:

- underweight (less than 18.5)
- normal (between 18.5 and 24.99)
- overweight (between 25 and 29.99)
- obese (30 and over).

There are further sub-classifications of obese BMIs that do not apply to the study cohort. Also, none of the players in the study cohort are in the underweight BMI category and only 3 players are obese. When BMI is analyzed as a categorical variable, these 3 players will be aggregated with the overweight group. Therefore, only 2 of the 4 BMI categories, normal and overweight, will be utilized in this study. The BMI categories are clinically meaningful, but continuous BMI may be more exact as no information is lost. Depending on the analysis, categorical and/or continuous BMI will be used.

4.7.3 Number of Career Years Played in Major League Baseball

A player is credited as participating in 1 year of Major League Baseball for each regular season that he played 1 or more games. Number of career years played Major League Baseball is a continuous variable. However, to make the results more comprehensible, ordered categories of this variable will also be created and used in the analysis as follows:

- 1–2 years
- 3–5 years
- 6–9 years
- 10–14 years
- 15 years or more.

4.7.4 Player Position

Player position is aggregated for the analysis in 2 ways. First, a dichotomous classification of pitchers and non-pitchers is created. Second, players are placed into one of the following 5 groups:

- catchers
- pitchers
- infielders
- outfielders
- other.

Infielders encompass first, second and third basemen, plus shortstops. Outfielders include right-, left- and center- fielders. The "other" position category includes designated hitters, pinch-runners, and pinch-hitters. When individuals play more than a single position, the position played in the most games is used in the analyses.

4.7.5 US Birthplace Region

Four US regions, i.e., Northeast, Midwest, South and West, are designated by the Census (US Census Bureau 2015) and are used by the CDC and other government agencies and organizations. Figure 4.1 contains a map of the US with each of the 4 regions color-coded. Birthplace region, or the region of the US where players are born, cannot be fully examined when Hispanics are included in the analyses. This is because all Hispanics in this study are, by definition, born in Latin American countries.

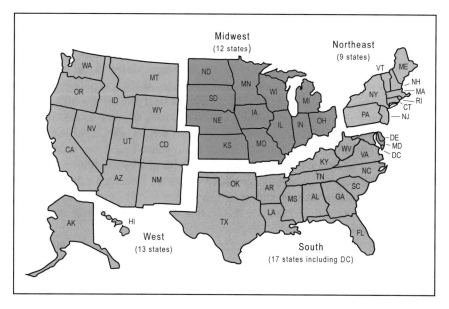

Fig. 4.1 Census regions and divisions of the United States

4.7.6 Handedness

In baseball, handedness can be defined in terms of the hand used to throw and the side used to bat. A player can bat from the right or left side of home plate and can also switch-hit, i.e., bat from either side of home plate. Hence, two handedness variables are formed based on throwing arm and batting side respectively.

4.8 Statistical Plan

This section details the statistical plan that will be used to describe the study cohort and to test the main study hypotheses. The analytic strategy will also include systematic testing of other independent variables. The empirical analysis will begin in Chap. 5 by describing the study cohort and examining the relationship between race/Hispanic origin and variables related to births and deaths, specifically year of birth and vital status. In addition, separate cross-tabulations of race/Hispanic origin by the year of birth categories and vital status will be accompanied by chi-square tests. Chap. 5 will conclude with a Cox proportional hazards regression that examines the year of birth categories in relation to all-cause mortality.

One of the key statistics derived from Cox regressions is the hazard ratio. This statistic reflects the risk of experiencing the event of interest, i.e., all-cause mortality, for the 3 groups of players, and can also contain other independent variables and covariates. Index referencing is a procedure that can be used in Cox models to determine mortality risk (based on hazard ratios) relative to a given group. As a hypothetical example, suppose overweight BMI players are being compared to normal weight individuals on mortality risk. The normal weight players could be assigned as the index reference and given a value of 0, while the overweight players would be given a value of 1. In this example, the hazard ratio would provide the estimated risk of dying for the overweight group using the normal weight group as the reference. For readers familiar with odds ratios, hazard ratios can be interpreted in a similar manner. For example, a hazard ratio of 1.75 in the hypothetical example, would indicate that overweight players have a 75% increased risk of all-cause mortality relative to normal BMI players. A hazard ratio that is less than 1 denotes a decreased risk of the outcome of interest. Continuing with the hypothetical example, a hazard ratio of 0.6 would reflect a 40% decreased risk of all-cause mortality for the overweight BMI group relative to those with a normal BMI.

The testing of the main study hypotheses related to mortality risk among the 3 race/Hispanic origin groups of players will be accomplished using a multi-level approach beginning with preliminary tests provided in Chap. 6. Comparisons will show vital status by race/Hispanic origin for all year of birth categories. Chapter 6 will conclude with a Cox model that tests whether mortality risk varies by race/Hispanic origin controlling for year of birth.

Assuming a statistical relationship between race/Hispanic origin and mortality (controlling for year of birth), the next step in the analytic process will be to examine additional independent variables to determine whether they add to the prediction of mortality risk. Alternatively, these other variables could be distorting relationships between race/Hispanic origin and mortality. This examination will engender at least 2 tests of significance to determine whether there is a relationship between each of the additional independent variables and:

1. race/Hispanic origin (using chi-square tests) and
2. mortality risk (using Cox models).

This latter test will control for year of birth and assess the relationship between each of these variables and all-cause mortality. If significant relationships are uncovered in both tests, then race/Hispanic origin will be added to the Cox model above.

In the final, most definitive testing of the study hypotheses, all the significant variables will be included along with race/Hispanic origin and year of birth in a multivariate Cox proportional hazards regression (Chap. 9). This test will indicate whether race/Hispanic origin persists as a predictor of mortality when all the significant study variables are controlled simultaneously.

The analyses described thus far are "internal" since they compare different groups of players within the study cohort. Chap. 10 will describe "external" analyses that separately compare mortality rates of players within the 3 race/Hispanic origin groups with gender- and, age-matched controls from the general population. Details on the statistical plan for the external analyses will be provided separately in Chap. 10.

Many statistical tests will be conducted in this book using an alpha level of 5% and no correction to this level will be made. Because of this, some false positive findings are likely. Readers are cautioned about this possibility.

4.9 SAS Procedures

The data analysis for this book will use SAS/BASE and SAS/STAT software, Version 9.4 of the SAS System for Windows 10 (SAS Institute Inc. 2018). The specific SAS procedures to be used include: Proc FREQ for frequency distributions and cross tabulations, Proc UNIVARIATE for descriptive statistics and histograms, Proc ANOVA for analysis of variance, Proc GLM for analysis of covariance, Proc PHREG for Cox proportional hazards regressions, and Proc STDRATE to obtain Standardized Mortality Ratios (SAS Institute Inc. 2018).

References

Allison, P. D. (2010). *Survival analysis using SAS: A practical guide* (2nd ed.). Cary: SAS Institute Inc.

Ashe, A., Jr. (1993). *A hard road to glory: The African-American athlete in basketball.* New York: Amistad Press.

Baseball Almanac. (2018). *MLB players by year of death.* Retrieved from http://www.baseball-almanac.com/players/baseball_deaths.php.

Cox, D. R., & Oakes, D. (1984). *Analysis of survival data.* New York: Chapman & Hall.

Find-a-Grave.com (2017). Retrieved from https://www.findagrave.com.

Lahman Baseball Database. (2017). *College playing spreadsheet.* Retrieved from http://www.seanlahman.com/baseball-archive/statistics/.

Lawler, T., Lawler, F., Gibson, J., & Murray, R. (2012). Does the African-American-white mortality gap persist after playing professional basketball? A 50-year historical cohort study. *Annals of Epidemiology, 22,* 406–412.

Los Angeles Times. (2017). *Obituaries database.* Retrieved from http://obituaries.latimes.com/category/sports/1/.

Markowitz, J. S. (2016). *Lost seasons: Arrests, suspensions, career chaos and mortality among National Football League (NFL) players.* North Charleston: CreateSpace.

Markowitz, J. S. (2018). *Mortality and its risk factors among professional athletes: A comparison between former NBA and NFL players.* Cham: Springer Nature.

SABR a, Society for American Baseball Research, (no date). *A guide to sabermetric research: How to find raw data.* Retrieved from https://sabr.org/sabermetrics/data.

SABR b, Society for American Baseball Research, (no date). *SABR baseball biography project.* Retrieved from http://sabr.org/bioproject.

SAS Institute Inc. (2018). *SAS/BASE and SAS/STATS, Version 9.4.* Cary: SAS Institute Inc.

Social Security Administration. (no date). *Actuarial Life Table.* Table entitled "Period Life Table, 2014". Retrieved from https://www.ssa.gov/oact/STATS/table4c6.html.

Sporting News. (2017). *Notable sports deaths of 2016.* Retrieved from http://www.sportingnews.com/other-sports/photos/notable-sports-deaths-of-2016-nfl-football-nba-basketball-baseball/e5dyl44gj40h1hbeq6bu9pm0o.

Sports Reference LLC. (2018). *Players pages.* Retrieved from https://www.baseball-reference.com/leagues/MLB/1960-opening-day-rosters.shtml.

Stewart, M., & Kennedy, M. (2002). *Hispanic baseball's finest fielders.* Brookfield: Twenty-First Century Books.

Tributes. (2017). *Celebrity deaths in sports.* Retrieved from http://www.tributes.com/celebrity/deaths/Sports.

US Census Bureau. (2015). *Geographic terms and concepts—Census divisions and census regions*. Retrieved from https://www.census.gov/geo/reference/gtc/gtc_census_divreg.html.

Wikipedia. (2018). *List of first Major League Baseball players*. Retrieved from https://en.wikipedia.org/wiki/List_of_first_black_Major_League_Baseball_players.

W.H.O. (World Health Organization). (2008). *BMI classification*. Retrieved from http://apps.who.int/bmi/index.jsp?introPage=intro_3.html.

Chapter 5
Births and Deaths in the Study Cohort

5.1 Results

5.1.1 Cohort Description

A total of 5263 former players who played Major League Baseball anytime between 1947 and 1986 are included in the analysis consisting of 4258 non-Hispanic whites (80.9%), 587 African-Americans (11.2%), and 418 Hispanics (7.9%). A total of 2018 of these 5263 former players (38.3%) died, while 3245 (61.7%) were still alive as of January 1, 2018. The mean and median year birth for the entire cohort is 1941.1 and 1943 respectively. This indicates that players still alive on the vital status end-date of January 1, 2018 average about 77–79 years of age.

5.1.2 Year of Birth by Race/Hispanic Origin

See Table 5.1 for a description of race/Hispanic origin and both the categorical and continuous versions of year of birth. The percentages of players born within each year of birth category are displayed, followed by mean and median year of birth for the 3 race/Hispanic origin groups. Clearly, non-Hispanic whites have an earlier year of birth compared to African-American and Hispanic players. This is confirmed by the significant overall test results for the comparisons of race/Hispanic origin for both the categorical and continuous versions of year of birth (p's < 0.0001). There are much higher percentages of non-Hispanic white players born in the earliest year of birth categories. For example, nearly 1 in 5 (18.2%) non-Hispanic white players are born prior to 1925 compared to less than 4% of African-Americans and 6.3% of Hispanics. For the more recent year of birth categories, the reverse pattern is evident; more than two-thirds of African-American players (67%) are born between 1945 and 1966 compared to 56.7% of Hispanics and only 42.5% of non-Hispanic

Table 5.1 Year of birth by race/Hispanic origin

Year of birth	Race/Hispanic origin						
	African-American		Hispanic		Non-Hispanic white		p-value*
	N	%	N	%	N	%	
1905–1914	2	0.3	6	1.4	122	2.9	<0.0001
1915–1924	21	3.6	20	4.8	655	15.4	
1925–1934	58	9.9	59	14.1	818	19.2	
1935–1944	113	19.3	96	23.0	855	20.1	
1945–1954	207	35.3	114	27.3	1010	23.7	
1955–1966	186	31.7	123	29.4	798	18.7	
Totals[a]	587	100.1	418	100.0	4258	100.0	
Mean/median year of birth	1947.8/1950		1945.6/1948		1939.7/1941		<0.0001

*Based on 3 × 6 chi-square test for categories and one way ANOVA for mean year of birth
[a]Total percentage may exceed 100% due to rounding

whites. Mean and median year of birth is also different for the 3 race/Hispanic origin groups. The mean year of birth for non-Hispanic white players is 1939.7 compared to 1947.8 for African-Americans and 1945.6 for Hispanics. Median year of birth differs by nine years between non-Hispanic whites (median = 1941) and African Americans (median = 1950). These differences in year of birth among the 3 study groups underscore the need to control for this variable in the statistical analyses of mortality risk.

5.1.3 Unadjusted Analysis of Vital Status by Race/Hispanic Origin

The year of birth results in the preceding paragraph increase the likelihood that a higher percentage of non-Hispanic white players died compared to the other 2 groups simply because they were older. As illustrated in Table 5.2, this turns out to be the case. In analyses *unadjusted* for year of birth, more than 40% of non-Hispanic white players have passed away compared to 32.1% of Hispanics and 26.9% of African-Americans.

Table 5.2 Vital status by race/Hispanic origin

Vital status	Race/Hispanic origin						p-value*
	African-American		Hispanic		Non-Hispanic white		
	N	%	N	%	N	%	
Alive	429	73.1	284	67.9	2532	59.5	<0.0001
Dead	158	26.9	134	32.1	1726	40.5	

*Based on 3 × 2 chi-square test

5.1.4 Vital Status by Race/Hispanic Origin Adjusted for Year of Birth

A Cox proportional hazards regression of the year of birth categories predicting mortality risk without controlling for any other variables is conducted. (These data are not shown in a table display.) Keeping in mind that the reference category for this analysis is the group of players born between 1955 and 1966, individuals born in the earliest year of birth group, i.e., 1905–1914, have a hazard ratio of 3.61, which is significant ($p < 0.0001$). These results mean that players born between 1905 and 1914 have a 3.6-fold increased risk of dying relative to those born between 1955 and 1966. As expected, the hazard ratios decline with each more proximate year of birth category, although these ratios (relative to the index group) continue to be significant for players in every age category. The hazard ratio is 3.44 for players born between 1915 and 1924 ($p < 0.0001$); 2.78 for players born between 1925 and 1934 ($p < 0.0001$); 2.11 for players born between 1935 and 1944 ($p < 0.0001$); and 1.74 for players born between 1945 and 1954 ($p = 0.0015$). Using the continuous version of year of birth also yields significant results ($p < 0.0001$). As expected, these results indicate that age, measured by year of birth, and mortality risk are inversely related.

5.1.5 Vital Status by Race/Hispanic Origin Stratified by Year of Birth

Table 5.3 depicts the percentage of players alive and dead, i.e., vital status, categorized by the 3 race/Hispanic origin groups and stratified by the 6 year of birth categories. During the earliest year of birth category, 1905–1914, all players in all 3 race/Hispanic origin groups have passed away. While there are 122 non-Hispanic whites born in this age category, only 2 African-Americans and 6 Hispanics were born in the designated period. Even in the next more proximate year of birth category, 1915–1924, there are limited numbers of survivors. Two of 21 African-Americans (9.5%), none of the 20 Hispanics (0%), and 22 of the 655 non-Hispanic whites (3.4%) born between 1915 and 1924 are still alive. The next year of birth category, 1925–1934, is different from the remaining more recent categories since there is a higher percentage of

Table 5.3 Vital status by year of birth categories and race/Hispanic origin

Year of birth	Race/Hispanic origin						
	African-American		Hispanic		Non-Hispanic white		p-value*
	N dead/N total	% dead	N dead/N total	% dead	N dead/N total	% dead	
1905–1914	2/2	100.0	6/6	100.0	122/122	100.0	n/a
1915–1924	19/21	90.5	20/20	100.0	633/655	96.6	0.2167
1925–1934	39/58	67.2	36/59	61.0	584/818	71.4	0.206
1935–1944	45/113	39.8	38/96	39.6	256/855	29.9	0.0249
1945–1954	40/207	19.3	25/114	21.9	111/1010	11.0	<0.0001
1955–1966	13/186	7.0	9/123	7.3	20/798	2.5	0.0015

*Based on 6 separate 3×2 chi-square tests

non-Hispanic whites who have passed away (71.4%) relative to African-Americans (67.2%) and Hispanics (61%). Beginning with the 1935–1944 year of birth category, there are significant vital status differences among the 3 race/Hispanic origin groups. In all these instances, there is a lower percentage of non-Hispanic white players who have passed away compared to African-Americans and Hispanics. These latter 2 groups have very similar percentages of players who have died in the more proximate year of birth categories. For example, within players born between 1945 and 1954, 19.3 and 21.9% of African-American and Hispanic players have died respectively compared to only 11% of non-Hispanic white players ($p < 0.0001$).

5.2 Summary of Results

- Year of birth varies significantly among the 3 race/Hispanic origin groups; non-Hispanic whites tend to be born in earlier year of birth categories indicating older ages.
- Unadjusted vital status by race/Hispanic origin results are misleading owing to the markedly different year of birth distributions of the 3 groups.
- Both the categorical and continuous versions of year of birth predict mortality risk in the expected direction; as year of birth is earlier, and age is increased, mortality risk is higher.
- Vital status by race/Hispanic origin results stratified by year of birth categories reveal several differences favoring non-Hispanic whites beginning in players born between 1935 and 1944 and continuing through 1955–1966.

In the next chapter, a preliminary test of the study hypotheses is described that considers time to all-cause mortality (rather than vital status) as the dependent variable. The analyses of independent variables other than race/Hispanic origin will follow in Chaps. 7 and 8.

Chapter 6
Preliminary Testing of Main Study Hypotheses

6.1 Introduction

Because the non-Hispanic whites in the study cohort tend to be older than players in the other 2 groups, *unadjusted* analyses of race/Hispanic origin by vital status described in Chap. 5 provide misleading results. However, after these results are stratified by year of birth categories, the mortality results become somewhat clearer. Within the younger players in the study cohort, compared to non-Hispanic white players, a higher percentage of African-Americans and Hispanics have died. However, no formal testing of the study hypotheses has been performed that treats all-cause mortality as a time-to-event variable and controls for a more precise (continuous) version of year of birth.

The next step in the analytic process is to conduct preliminary testing of the main study hypotheses regarding race/Hispanic origin and mortality risk. The results presented in this chapter remain preliminary since only year of birth is controlled in the analysis. If the preliminary results are significant, the goal of the remaining analyses will be to identify other variables that may affect the relationship between race/Hispanic origin and mortality. These other variables may also add independently to the prediction of mortality risk, above and beyond what is already explained by race/Hispanic origin. The last step of the analysis will be to re-test the main study hypotheses while controlling for *all* the significant variables simultaneously.

J. S. Markowitz, *Mortality Among Hispanic and African-American Players After Desegregation in Major League Baseball*, SpringerBriefs in Public Health, https://doi.org/10.1007/978-3-030-17280-0_6

6.2 Empirical Results

6.2.1 Testing of Differences in Mortality Risk Based on Race/Hispanic Origin

Table 6.1 shows the results of Cox proportional hazards regressions predicting time to all-cause mortality risk using (continuous) year of birth as a covariate with race/Hispanic origin as an independent class variable. Year of birth is a significant negative covariate of mortality risk ($p < 0.0001$). This means that as players get older, predictably, their risk of dying increases.

Table 6.1 also indicates that compared to non-Hispanic white players, mortality risk is significantly elevated among African-Americans (hazard ratio $= 1.38$; $p = 0.0001$) and Hispanics (hazard ratio $= 1.21$; $p = 0.0398$). In other words, controlling solely for year of birth, African-Americans have a 38% increased risk of mortality compared to non-Hispanic whites, and Hispanics have a 21% increased risk. With Hispanic players as the index reference, African-Americans have an increased mortality risk of about 15% that is not statistically significant ($p = 0.2498$). Because African-Americans have the highest mortality risk of the 3 race/Hispanic origin groups, when they serve as the index reference group, the hazard ratios for the other 2 groups are less than 1, reflecting protection against mortality for non-Hispanic whites and Hispanics. That is, compared to African-Americans, non-Hispanic white players have about a 28% decreased risk of mortality that's significant and Hispanics have about a 13% decreased risk that is not significant.

Table 6.1 Cox proportional hazards regressions predicting mortality risk by race/Hispanic origin controlling for year of birth with rotating index reference groups

Variables	Hazard ratio	p-value	Hazard ratio	p-value	Hazard ratio	p-value
Year of birth (continuous)	0.97	<0.0001	0.97	<0.0001	0.97	<0.0001
Race/Hispanic origin						
African-American	1.38	0.0001	1.15	0.2498	Index reference	
Hispanic	1.21	0.0398	Index reference		0.87	0.2498
Non-Hispanic white	Index reference		0.83	0.0398	0.72	0.0001

6.2.2 Summary of Empirical Results

- With year of birth controlled in Cox regressions, non-Hispanic white players have significantly lower mortality risk compared to both African-Americans and Hispanics. Mortality risk is highest among African-American players.
- There is no significant difference in mortality risk between Hispanic and African-American players when only year of birth is controlled.

The results presented in this chapter provide preliminary support for the hypothesis that: compared to non-Hispanic white players, African-Americans are disadvantaged when it comes to mortality risk. In addition, former Hispanic players also have elevated mortality risk compared to non-Hispanic whites, although this result is marginally significant. There is a need to further identify other variables that can be included in additional regression analyses to help confirm or refute these preliminary results.

Part III
Other Independent Variables and More Definitive Testing of Study Hypotheses

Chapter 7
The Role of Educational Attainment

7.1 Education, Race, and National Origin

The education of children represents a fundamental resource for both individuals and the larger society since it shapes life chances. Unfortunately, in the US, there has never been a level playing field between the races when it comes to education. Through the years, discriminatory laws and policies have impeded the education of African-Americans. The landmark 1954 Supreme Court decision in the Brown versus Board of Education case declared segregation in schools to be unconstitutional. Real integration of schools, however, failed to materialize for at least 10 years after the Brown decision (Klarman 1994), and even then, African–American access to schools on par with whites has been elusive (Orfield and Frankenberg 2014).

One of the cornerstones of the Civil Rights Movement of the 1960s involves education. Title VI of the Civil Rights Act of 1964 prohibits discrimination based on race, color or national origin. While substantial progress in education has occurred since the Civil Rights Act was enacted (US Department of Education 1999), the level of accomplishment falls short as it fails to effectively deal with residential segregation and its impact on education. African-Americans often reside in high-poverty communities, and because of this frequently attend public schools in communities with predominantly African-American students. Since school resources in the US are often allocated in an uneven manner based on race (Boozer et al. 1992), schools attended mainly by African-American students receive fewer resources than those attended by whites (US Commission on Civil Rights 2018).

A brief overview of education statistics in the US general population will be provided in the next section. This will be followed by some of the available educational statistics related to the Hispanic cohort countries. More than 85% of the African-Americans and over 62% of the non-Hispanic whites in the current study cohort were born sometime between 1935 and 1966. Consequently, most of them attended primary and secondary school between 1940 and 1970. For this reason, the section that follows focuses on US education statistics for this period.

© The Author(s), under exclusive license to Springer Nature Switzerland AG 2019
J. S. Markowitz, *Mortality Among Hispanic and African-American Players After Desegregation in Major League Baseball*, SpringerBriefs in Public Health,
https://doi.org/10.1007/978-3-030-17280-0_7

7.2   Historical Educational Attainment Statistics by Race/Hispanic Origin

Median years of school completed by residents of US and Hispanic cohort country males aged 25 and older for the years 1940, 1950, 1960 and 1970 are summarized in Table 7.1. (These published reports use "whites" and "Blacks" to describe the 2 US races.) In 1940, US whites complete 8.7 years of school compared to 5.4 years for blacks. This 3-year difference in years of school completed generally continues in subsequent decades addressed with medians of 9.3 and 6.4 years for whites and blacks respectively in 1950; 10.6 and 7.9 years respectively in 1960; and 12.2 and 9.4 years respectively in 1970. Encouragingly, these data reveal that the number of school years completed increases substantially between 1940 and 1970 for both races. Nevertheless, the educational gap between the races persists over the 30-year period covered in Table 7.1.

The median number of school years completed indicate very large differences for male youths in Hispanic cohort countries compared to the US. In 1940 and 1950, the median number of school years completed generally average about 1, 2 or, at most 3.7 years for males living in Hispanic cohort countries aged 25 years and over. In 1960, males complete a median of 3–4 years of school in the Hispanic cohort countries, and in 1970 the median rises to about 4–7 years. The pattern of the statistics shown in Table 7.1 indicates improvement in educational attainment in the Hispanic cohort countries between 1940 and 1970, although the median years of school completed are far below averages reported in the US.

In summary, in the US general population, African–American students achieve lower levels of educational attainment than whites between 1940 and 1970. However, educational attainment among students in the Hispanic cohort countries is far lower than in the US.

7.3   Education and Mortality in the Scientific Literature

Attention now turns to the relationship between education and mortality which has been found to be statistically related in numerous general population studies (Grossman and Kaestner 1997; Xu et al. 2010; Rogers et al. 2000; National Center for Health Statistics 2012). For example, Xu and colleagues (2010) determined that death rates in the US in 2007 are about 2.5 times higher for individuals who fail to graduate high school compared to those with some college education. In another study that examines life expectancy at age 25, the group of individuals with college degrees live about 10 years longer than those who do not have a high school degree (National Center for Health Statistics 2012). There is also empirical evidence that the association between mortality and education persists even when other elements of socioeconomic status, like income and occupation, are statistically controlled (Grossman and Kaestner 1997; Rogers et al. 2000). Several researchers have concluded that the relationship between education and mortality is causal (Llleras-Muney 2002; Rogers et al. 2000). The Hispanic Paradox (see Chap. 3) represents a possible exception to the well-established relationship between education and mortality.

Table 7.1 Median number of school years completed in US by race and Hispanic cohort countries, 1940–1970 (males aged 25 years and older)

Race (US) and Hispanic cohort countries	Year			
	1940	1950	1960	1970
United States	Median years of school completed			
White	8.7	9.3	10.6	12.2
Black[a]	5.4	6.4	7.9	9.4
Hispanic cohort countries				
Colombia	2.7	2.5	3.6	5.0
Cuba	3.4	3.6	4.1	6.3
Dominican Republic	2.1	2.3	3.4	4.6
Mexico	3.3	2.4	3.1	4.3
Nicaragua	1.4	1.5	3.5	5.1
Panama	3.7	4.3	5.3	5.7
Venezuela	1.2	2.0	3.2	5.1
Puerto Rico[*]	n/a	3.7	4.6	6.9

[a]Between 1940 and 1960, Blacks include persons of "other" races
US data
Source U.S. Department of Commerce, Bureau of the Census, Historical Statistics of the United States, Colonial Times to 1970; Current Population Series, p. 20, Educational Attainment of the United States Population, various years; and "Education of the American Population," by John K. Folger and Charles B. Nam, prepared in 1998. Located at: https://nces.ed.gov/pubs93/93442.pdf, Table 5
Hispanic cohort country data
Sources Barro-Lee Educational Attainment Dataset
Educational Attainment for Male Population Aged 15–24, 1870–2010
Located at: http://Www.barrolee.com/
Barro, Robert and Jong-Wha Lee, 2013, "A New Data Set o f Educational Attainment in the World, 1950–2010." Journal of Development Economics, vol. 104, pp. 184–198
[*]Separate data source for males in Puerto Rico. Data applies to "adult population"
Located at: http://Www.columbia.edu/~flr9/documents/Ladd_Rivera_Batiz_%20Education_ Development.pdf
Ladd, H.F. and Rivera-Batiz, F.L. Education and Economic Development. The Economy of Puerto Rico: Restoring Growth, edited by SM Collins, BP Bosworth and MA Soto-Class Brookings Institution Press, 2007, Washington DC, Fig. 5.1

7.4 Empirical Results

The primary goal of the analysis described in this chapter is to determine the role that education plays with respect to race/Hispanic origin as well as mortality. It has already been documented in Chap. 6 that among former Major League Baseball players, race/Hispanic origin is statistically related to mortality risk controlling for year of birth. How will the inclusion of education in the analysis impact on the relationship between race/Hispanic origin and mortality?

7.4.1 Educational Attainment and Race/Hispanic Origin

As shown in Table 7.2, there are significant differences between race/Hispanic origin and educational attainment (p < 0.0001). Consistent with general population statistics provided earlier, Hispanic players are the least educated of the 3 race/Hispanic origin groups. More than three-quarters of Hispanic players have little or no high school education compared to only 8% of African-Americans and 12.9% of non-Hispanic whites. Just over 20% of Hispanics have at least some high school education and less than 4% have any kind of college education. Nearly half of all African-American players and more than 56% of non-Hispanic whites have at least some college education.

Table 7.2 Educational attainment of Major League Baseball players by race/Hispanic origin

| Educational attainment | Race/Hispanic origin | | | | | | p-value[a] |
| | African-Americans | | Hispanics | | Non-Hispanic whites | | |
	N	%	N	%	N	%	
Little or no high school	47	8.0	316	75.6	548	12.9	<0.0001
At least some high school, but no college	250	42.6	86	20.6	1303	30.6	
Some college, but unknown number of years completed	85	14.5	6	1.4	631	14.8	
1–2 years of college completed	96	16.4	4	1.0	817	19.2	
3 or more years of college completed	109	18.6	6	1.4	959	22.5	

[a]Based on 3 × 5 chi-square test

Variables	Hazard ratio	p-value
Year of birth (continuous)	0.98	<0.0001
Educational attainment		
Little or no high school	1.59	<0.0001
At least some high school, but no college	1.36	0.0001
Some college, but unknown number of years completed	1.17	0.0807
1–2 years of college completed	1.11	0.2645
3 or more years of college completed	Index reference	

Table 7.3 Cox proportional hazards regression predicting mortality risk based on educational attainment controlling for year of birth

7.4.2 Educational Attainment and Mortality Risk

Educational attainment is also associated with mortality risk controlling for (continuous) year of birth. See Table 7.3. The highest level of educational attainment captured in this study, players with 3 or more years of college, serves as the index reference group for the Cox regression analysis, which examines mortality risk based on educational attainment controlling for year of birth. Compared to players with the most education, the hazard ratios for all other educational attainment levels exceed unity and increase in magnitude with consecutively lower levels of education. For example, players with the lowest levels of education, i.e., little or no high school, have a 59% increased risk of dying compared to those with the most education (p < 0.0001). For the next least educated group (with at least some high school), the hazard ratio of 1.36 is also significant (p = 0.0001).

7.4.3 Does Educational Attainment Affect the Relationship Between Race/Hispanic Origin and Mortality Risk?

Table 7.4 contains a Cox regression predicting mortality risk that includes race/Hispanic origin and educational attainment while controlling for year of birth. Like the analysis that examines mortality differences among the 3 race/Hispanic origin groups described in Chap. 6, African-American players continue to be at elevated risk compared to non-Hispanic whites when educational attainment is added to the analysis with a hazard ratio of 1.35 (p < 0.0001). The results for Hispanics, however, change when educational attainment is controlled. In the analysis presented in Table 6.1 that control for year of birth but do not include educational attainment, the hazard ratio is 1.21 which is marginally significant for Hispanics compared to non-Hispanic whites (p = 0.0398). When educational attainment is added to this

Table 7.4 Cox proportional hazards regression predicting mortality risk based on educational attainment and race/Hispanic origin controlling for year of birth

Variables	Hazard ratio	p-value
Year of birth (continuous)	0.98	<0.0001
Race/Hispanic origin		
African-American	1.35	0.0005
Hispanic	0.98	0.8524
Non-Hispanic white	Index reference	
Educational attainment		
Little or no high school	1.59	<0.0001
At least some high school, but no college	1.36	0.0001
Some college, but unknown number of years completed	1.17	0.0875
1–2 years of college completed	1.12	0.2378
3 or more years of college completed	Index reference	

analysis in Table 7.4, mortality risk for Hispanic players is about the same as non-Hispanic whites (hazard ratio = 0.98) and is no longer significant (p = 0.8524). Furthermore, this analysis indicates that African-American players are at significant mortality risk compared to Hispanics (hazard ratio = 1.37; p = 0.0102). (data not shown) Again, this result is substantively different from the one previously obtained that does not control for educational attainment and has a hazard ratio = 1.15 which is not significant.

Hispanics are no longer at elevated mortality risk compared to non-Hispanic whites when education is controlled in the analysis. Additional multivariate analyses are required to determine whether this attenuating effect of race/Hispanic origin on mortality persists when all other significant variables are simultaneously controlled. Given the very skewed distribution of educational attainment among Hispanic players, this result could be a statistical anomaly. Post hoc stratified analyses are also required to help confirm or refute these findings.

7.5   Summary of Empirical Results

- Educational attainment varies significantly by race/Hispanic origin. Hispanic players are easily the least educated of the 3 groups.
- Overall, mortality risk increases significantly as educational attainment decreases.
- When included in the analysis, educational attainment equalizes the risk of mortality between Hispanic and non-Hispanic white players.

- The distribution of educational attainment among Hispanic players is highly skewed toward very low levels. This could distort the statistical results.

References

Boozer, M. A., Kruger, A. B. & Wolkon, S. (1992). Race and school quality since Brown vs. Board of Education. *Brookings Paper on Economic Activity: Microeconomics*. Retrieved from: https://www.brookings.edu/wp-content/uploads/1992/01/1992_bpeamicro_boozer.pdf.

Grossman, M., & Kaestner, R. (1997). Effects of education on health. In J. R. Berhman & N. Stacey (Eds.), *The social benefits of education*. Ann Arbor: University of Michigan Press.

Klarman, M. J. (1994). How Brown changed race relations. *The Journal of American History, 81*(1), 81–118.

Lleras-Muney, A. (2002). *The relationship between education and adult mortality in the United States, National Bureau of Education Research (NBER)* (Working Paper No. 8696). Retrieved from http://www.nber.org/papers/w8986.pdf.

National Center for Health Statistics. (2012). *Health, United States, 2011: With Special Feature on Socioeconomic Status and Health*, Figure 32. Retrieved from: https://www.cdc.gov/nchs/data/hus/hus11.pdf.

Orfield, G. & Frankenberg, E. (2014). Brown at 60. The Civil Rights project. Retrieved from https://civilrightsproject.ucla.edu/research/k-12-education/integration-and-diversity/brown-at-60-great-progress-a-long-retreat-and-an-uncertain-future/Brown-at-60-051814.pdf.

Rogers, R. G., Robert A. Hummer, R. A., & Nam, C. B. (2000). *Living and Dying in the USA*. Cambridge: Academic Press.

US Commission on Civil Rights (2018). Public education funding inequity. Retrieved from https://www.usccr.gov/pubs/2018/2018-01-10-Education-Inequity.pdf.

US Department of Education (1999). Office for Civil Rights. Impact of the Civil Rights laws. Retrieved from https://www2.ed.gov/about/offices/list/ocr/docs/impact.html.

Xu, J., Kochanek, K. D., Murphy, S. L., & Tejada-Vera, B. (2010). Deaths: Final data for 2007. *National Vital Statistics Reports, 58,* 1–73.

Chapter 8
Examination of Other Independent Variables

8.1 Introduction

Preliminary empirical results presented in Chap. 6 indicate that non-Hispanic white Major League Baseball players are at decreased mortality risk compared to Hispanic and especially African-American players. Chapter 7 results indicate that educational attainment and mortality risk are inversely related. In addition, educational attainment mediates differences in mortality risk between Hispanic and non-Hispanic white players. Five other independent variables will be examined in this chapter; BMI, US birthplace region, total years played Major League Baseball, player position and handedness.

Statistical associations between these variables and race/Hispanic origin and all-cause mortality could indicate that these other variables are themselves, risk or protective factors for mortality. Such associations may also attenuate or strengthen the relationship between race/Hispanic origin and mortality risk.

Brief literature reviews of these 5 variables will be included in this chapter along with rationales for considering them in the analysis. When available, these literature reviews will focus on general populations as well as professional athletes. Items that add significantly to the prediction of mortality risk or alter the relationship between race/Hispanic origin described in Chap. 6 will be examined simultaneously in the multivariate analyses in Chap. 9.

8.2 Body Mass Index (BMI)

8.2.1 Background

The problem of obesity has been described in recent decades as an epidemic (Mitchell et al. 2011) with substantial public health ramifications. While estimates of the preva-

© The Author(s), under exclusive license to Springer Nature Switzerland AG 2019
J. S. Markowitz, *Mortality Among Hispanic and African-American Players After Desegregation in Major League Baseball*, SpringerBriefs in Public Health,
https://doi.org/10.1007/978-3-030-17280-0_8

lence of obesity in the US and elsewhere vary over time, it is hard to think of this issue as anything but a major worldwide problem affecting tens of millions of people. In one study of nearly 200 countries spanning a 25-year period, it was determined that "… excess body weight accounted for about 4 million deaths and 120 million disability-adjusted life-years worldwide in 2015" (GBD 2015 Obesity Collaborators 2017). In the US alone, as many as 2 out of every 3 adults are either overweight or obese (Berrington de Gonzalez et al. 2010). The idea that obesity could be a mutable risk factor that, if controlled, could reduce or eliminate select health problems, and perhaps even extend life, makes it a prime target for public health intervention. With its affordability and ease of administration, the BMI has become a global standard to help identify underweight, overweight and obese individuals; groups who may be at-risk for a variety of health conditions.

8.2.2 BMI and Race/Hispanic Origin in the General Population

BMI is believed to be associated with race/Hispanic origin and mortality in the general population. This relationship has been well documented in the scientific literature (Wagner and Heyward 2000; Deurenberg-Yap and Deurenberg 2003; Hsu et al. 2012; Flegal et al. 2002; Seo and Torabi 2006). According to the CDC, in the US general population, the age-adjusted prevalence of obesity among men in 2015–2016 averaged 37.9% for non-Hispanic whites, 36.9% for non-Hispanic blacks, and 43.1% for Hispanics (Hales et al. 2017). BMI's relationship with race/Hispanic origin generally comes from associations with SES. In general, SES and BMI are inversely related. According to one author: "People with more knowledge, money, power, prestige and beneficial social connections are better able to control weight gain, either through the ability to make healthy food choices … or through greater opportunities for exercise, and safe play" (Clarke et al. 2009).

8.2.3 BMI and Mortality in the General Population

Although the BMI measure was not developed specifically as a predictor of mortality risk, its relationship to many serious health problems, makes it useful for this purpose. The literature is equivocal, with respect to *overweight* (rather than obese) BMI since it is inconsistently related to negative health outcomes in general populations (Flegal et al. 2007). The more certain threats to health are linked to *obese* BMI levels. For example, obese BMI has been found to be related to things like coronary heart disease, stroke, type 2 diabetes, hypertension, stroke, gallbladder disease, several forms of cancer, osteoarthritis, and psychosocial problems (W.H.O. Fact Sheet 2016; CDC 2015; Hojjat and Hojatt 2017). Obese and sometimes overweight BMI may elevate mortality risk in general population studies (Prospective Studies Collaboration 2009; Kassirer and Angell 1998; Allison et al. 1999).

8.2.4 BMI and Professional Athletes

Several professional athlete studies have also documented the role of BMI as it relates to mortality (Baron and Rinsky 1994; Baron et al. 2012; Markowitz 2018; Lawler et al. 2012). But like the general population literature, the BMI level required to affect excess mortality risk is unclear. For some groups of professional athletes, like former NBA players, overweight BMI is adequate to lead to increased mortality risk. In other groups, like NFL players, obese BMI is required to raise the risk of dying (Markowitz 2018).

8.2.4.1 Professional Basketball Players

Because BMI fails to consider the amount of lean muscle mass (Nuttall 2015), there is some evidence that it may be flawed as a measurement tool, particularly when it comes to tall, buff athletes and other special groups. Markowitz (2018) found that the range of BMI scores among former basketball players was extremely limited and that no NBA players, of the 1398 studied, had obese scores. Both these findings seem anomalous given that NBA players average over 205 lb. Nevertheless, the tall heights of most basketball players reduce their chances of being classified as obese on BMI. In fact, only about 13% of NBA players reach the overweight plateau. Nevertheless, *overweight* BMI among NBA players is a significant independent predictor of all-cause mortality risk in multivariate analyses that control for other risk factors. Compared to normal weight NBA players, individuals with overweight BMIs have about a 50% increased risk of mortality (Markowitz 2018).

8.2.4.2 Professional Football Players

Baron and Rinsky (1994) report significant effects for BMI on cardiovascular mortality in their study of former NFL players. Controlling for race and several other variables, NFL players with BMI scores between 28 and 31 have more than 2.5 times the risk of dying compared to players with BMIs that are less than 28. This effect is more robust among players with the highest BMIs of 32 and over who have more than a 6-fold increased risk of cardiovascular deaths relative to players with lower scores (Baron and Rinsky 1994). A follow-up study of a sub-sample of these same NFL players conducted 17 years later provides significant results for obese (but not overweight) BMI predicting cardiovascular mortality (Baron et al. 2012). In one study, about 90% of NFL players who played any regular seasons between 1960 and 1986 had either overweight or obese BMI levels, and while overweight NFL players were not at significant increased risk of all-cause mortality, obese players were (Markowitz 2018).

8.3 Empirical Results

Only 3 of 5263 players in the current study cohort have BMIs in the obese range. These players are aggregated with overweight individuals when categorical BMI is analyzed.

8.3.1 BMI and Race/Hispanic Origin

See Table 8.1 for a cross-tabulation of race/Hispanic origin by the normal and overweight BMI categories included in this study. About 43% of both African-American and non-Hispanic white players have overweight BMIs. Hispanic players have lower BMIs with only 25.6% scoring in the overweight range. These differences are significant among the 3 race/Hispanic origin groups ($p < 0.0001$). Mean BMI is similar between African-American and non-Hispanic white players averaging about 24.6. However, Hispanic players have lower mean BMIs of 23.8. The overall test statistic comparing the 3 BMI means is significant ($p < 0.0001$).

8.3.2 BMI and Mortality Risk

See Table 8.2. Major League Baseball players with overweight BMIs have an 18% increased risk of mortality compared to normal BMI players after controlling for year of birth ($p = 0.0002$). Similar statistical results are obtained when continuous

Table 8.1 Categorical, mean and median BMI by race/Hispanic origin

BMI	Race/Hispanic origin						
	African-American		Hispanic		Non-Hispanic white		p-value*
	N	%	N	%	N	%	
Normal	334	56.9	307	73.4	2421	56.9	<0.0001
Overweight	253	43.1	111	26.6	1837	43.1	
Mean/median	24.6/24.4		23.8/23.7		24.7/24.4		<0.0001

*Based on 3×2 chi-square test for categories and oneway ANOVA for mean BMI

Table 8.2 Cox proportional hazard regression predicting mortality risk based on BMI controlling for year of birth

Variables	Hazard ratio	p-value
Year of birth (continuous)	0.98	<0.0001
BMI		
Normal	Index reference	
Overweight	1.18	0.0002

BMI is substituted for the 2 categories (p = 0.0008). Simply put, as BMI increases, so does mortality risk.

8.3.3 Does BMI Affect the Relationship Between Race/Hispanic Origin and Mortality Risk?

See Table 8.3, which in addition to controlling for year of birth, also contains terms for (categorical) BMI and race/Hispanic origin. With non-Hispanic whites as the reference group, both African-American and Hispanic players have significantly elevated risks of mortality with hazard ratios of 1.39 and 1.22 respectively (p's = 0.0001 and 0.0288). When the index reference group is Hispanics (data not shown), there is no significant difference between them and African-American players (hazard ratio = 1.14; p = 0.2831). In other words, controlling for year of birth and BMI, African-Americans and Hispanics have higher mortality risk than non-Hispanic whites but there is no significant difference between African-American and Hispanic players.

Table 8.3 Cox proportional hazards regression predicting mortality risk based on (categorical) BMI and race/Hispanic origin controlling for year of birth

Variables	Hazard ratio	p-value
Year of birth (continuous)	0.98	<0.0001
Race/Hispanic origin		
African-American	1.39	0.0001
Hispanic	1.22	0.0288
Non-Hispanic white	Index reference	
BMI		
Normal	Index reference	
Overweight	1.19	<0.0001

8.3.4   Summary of Empirical Results

- Almost no former Major League Baseball players have obese BMIs.
- About 43% of both non-Hispanic white and African-American players have over-weight BMIs compared to 26.6% of Hispanics.
- Players with overweight BMIs have a significant 18% increased risk of mortality compared to normal weight individuals.
- Overweight BMI continues to be a significant independent predictor of mortality risk when race/Hispanic origin is added to the analysis.
- With year of birth and BMI controlled, compared to non-Hispanic whites, mortality risk is significantly elevated among African-American and Hispanic players.

Despite its statistical relationship with both race/Hispanic origin and mortality risk, BMI adds independently to mortality in this study and can be considered a risk factor among former Major League Baseball players. Multivariate analyses are required to determine whether this pattern of results persists when other significant variables are controlled simultaneously. Moreover, the association between race/Hispanic origin and mortality does not change when BMI is added to the analysis.

8.4   US Birthplace Region

8.4.1   Background

Based on sociodemographic variables that are frequently related to SES, as well as a host of other factors, some areas or communities may be more likely to practice certain lifestyle-related behaviors (Diehr et al. 1993), experience lower or higher rates of specific diseases (Diez Roux 2001), and/or live shorter or longer lifespans (Yen and Kaplan 1999). Statistics on disease, death, and a range of health-related conditions among residents of large administrative units can be obtained at the aggregate level from a variety of organizations like the US Census Bureau (no date), the CDC (2018), and W.H.O. (2017).

When it comes to former professional athletes, data on birthplace, rather than current residence, is generally available. More than 90% of former professional basketball and football players attend high school in the same region where they are born (Markowitz 2018). This is meaningful because conditions and events experienced during childhood can have significant impacts on future health that can span a lifetime (Yen and Syme 1999). Because of its availability as well as its potential effect on health, US birthplace region will be examined in this chapter.

The investigation of mortality risk in professional athletes based on birthplace region has not received much attention. As far as I can tell, only 1 previous professional athlete study that includes NBA and NFL players has examined this relationship (Markowitz 2018). Being born in the South is a significant independent predictor of mortality among former NFL players, but this is not the case among former NBA players. Multivariate analyses that control for other risk factors reveal a significant 42% increase in mortality risk among NFL players born in the South compared to the West. No such relationship exists among former NBA players (Markowitz 2018). None of the previous Major League Baseball mortality studies have examined the role of residence or birthplace region.

A map of the US showing the 4 US regions has previously been displayed in Fig. 4.1.

8.5 Empirical Results

8.5.1 US Birthplace Region by Race

Again, Hispanic players are excluded from the analyses presented in this chapter.

See Table 8.4. There are significant differences between races with respect to the US birthplace region. More than 57% of African-American players are born in a Southern state compared to 27.6% of non-Hispanic whites (p < 0.0001). There are higher percentages of non-Hispanic whites born in the Midwest (28.2%) and the Northeast (21.4%) relative to African-Americans who average 14% and 8% respectively.

8.5.2 US Birthplace Region by Mortality Risk

See Table 8.5. Controlling for year of birth, players born in the South have a 17% increased risk of mortality compared to individuals born in the West (p = 0.0231).

Table 8.4 US birthplace region by race

US birthplace region	Race				
	African-American		Non-Hispanic white		p-value*
	N	%	N	%	
Midwest	82	14.0	1200	28.2	<0.0001
Northeast	47	8.0	909	21.4	
South	335	57.1	1175	27.6	
West	123	21.0	974	22.9	

Note Hispanics excluded from birthplace region analysis
*Based on 2 × 4 chi-square test

Table 8.5 Cox proportional hazards regression predicting mortality risk based on US birthplace region controlling for year of birth

Variables	Hazard ratio	p-value
Year of birth (continuous)	0.98	<0.0001
US birthplace region		
West	Index reference	
Midwest	1.06	0.4412
Northeast	1.0	0.9929
South	1.17	0.0231

Note Hispanics excluded from birthplace region analysis

8.5.3   Does US Birthplace Region Affect the Relationship Between Race and Mortality Risk?

Table 8.6 contains the results of a Cox proportional hazards regression predicting mortality risk based on race, US birthplace region and year of birth. While Southern birthplace region is significant in the previous analysis that excludes race, the hazard ratio is weakened by adding race to the model. The 17% increased risk (versus the Western region) drops to 13% and is no longer significant (p = 0.0862) when race is added.

8.5.4   Summary of Empirical Results

- A significantly larger percentage of African-American players are born in the South compared to non-Hispanic white players.
- Compared to the West, players born in the South have a significant 17% increased risk of mortality when only year of birth is controlled.
- When race is added to the analysis, it persists as a mortality predictor, but being born in the South is no longer a significant risk factor.

The empirical results indicate that any marginally significant association between birthplace region and mortality is likely to be a function of race. US birthplace region will be omitted from the multivariate assessments in Chap. 9 since its inclusion would eliminate Hispanics from the analyses and would make it impossible to test several study hypotheses.

Table 8.6 Cox proportional hazards regression predicting mortality risk based on US birthplace region and race controlling for year of birth

Variables	Hazard ratio	p-value
Year of birth (continuous)	0.97	<0.0001
US birthplace region		
West	Index reference	
Midwest	1.05	0.4722
Northeast	1.0	0.982
South	1.13	0.0862
Race		
African-American	1.35	0.0007
Non-Hispanic white	Index reference	

Note Hispanics excluded from US birthplace region analysis

8.6 Total Number of Years Played in Major League Baseball

8.6.1 Background

To play professional baseball, at least 3 things are necessary. First, players must be good enough at baseball to fend-off fierce competition from others. Second, serious injuries that reduce players' effectiveness and productivity must be avoided. Third, players must remain physically and mentally healthy, independent of play-related injuries. The length of careers may provide a measure of how well players fare with respect to these and other factors.

Salaries in baseball during the years covered in this study were not nearly as high as they are today (Badenhausen 2016). Yet compared to the general population of their time, Major League Baseball salaries between 1960 and 1986 are higher than the average general population salary during that period. For example, in 1970 the US average wage is $6,186 (Social Security Administration 2015) compared to Major League Baseball player salaries that average $29,303 (Shaikin 2016). By 1985, these same statistics get higher and more disparate; $16,823 for the general population (Social Security Administration 2015) and $371,157 for baseball players (Shaikin 2016). African-American and Hispanic player salaries are less than their non-Hispanic white counterparts in Major League Baseball (Scully 1973) and differences like these have been documented in other professional sports as well (Lawler et al. 2012). However, relative to their African-American and Hispanic peers in the general population, on average, players earn higher salaries. For players who are contracted by a Major League Baseball team for more than several years, the money adds-up over time and could influence SES. In turn, access to quality health care could be favorably impacted. In addition, life style decisions related to smoking, alcohol consumption and physical activity can be influenced by SES (Govil et al. 2009) and these behaviors can affect health and mortality.

8.6.2   Literature Review

The relationship between the length of professional players' careers and mortality has been studied several times. When an association between these variables is uncovered, it is inverse. This is the case with respect to professional basketball players (Lawler et al. 2012; Markowitz 2018), and Major League Baseball players (Saint Onge et al. 2008). Several studies, however, fail to uncover an inverse relationship (Abel and Kruger 2005). Also, no inverse relationship between career length and mortality is evident among former NFL players (Markowitz 2018).

8.7   Empirical Results

8.7.1   Total Years of Playing Experience and Race/Hispanic Origin

The top part of Table 8.7 contains a cross-tabulation of race/Hispanic origin by the categorical version of total number of career years of Major League Baseball playing experience. In general, Hispanic players have more years of experience relative to non-Hispanic whites. African-Americans have the most career playing experience relative to the other 2 groups (p < 0.0001). For example, about 37% of African-American players have 10 or more years of career playing experience compared to 28.7% of Hispanics and 27.3% of non-Hispanic whites. Comparisons of the mean and median number of career years played (see bottom of Table 8.7) confirm the categorical results.

Table 8.7 Total number of Major League Baseball years played by race/Hispanic origin

Total years played	Race/Hispanic origin						
	African-American		Hispanic		Non-Hispanic white		p-value*
	N	%	N	%	N	%	
1–2 years	125	21.3	111	26.6	1241	29.2	<0.0001
3–5 years	120	20.4	96	23.0	929	21.8	
6–9 years	125	21.3	91	21.8	926	21.8	
10–14 years	125	21.3	64	15.3	799	18.8	
15+ years	92	15.7	56	13.4	363	8.5	
Mean/median career years played	8.0/7.0		7.0/6.0		6.5/5.0		<0.0001

*Based on 3 × 5 chi-square test for categories and oneway ANOVA for mean BMI

8.7.2 Total Years of Playing Experience and Mortality Risk

See Table 8.8. Controlling for year of birth and using 1–2 total career years played as the index reference, only the players with the most Major League Baseball experience, i.e., 15 or more years, are significantly protected from mortality with a hazard ratio of 0.81 (p = 0.0193). However, the hazard ratios get smaller with each successive playing experience category beginning with individuals with 6–9 career years played (hazard ratio = 0.98, p = 0.753). Players with 10–14 years of experience have a hazard ratio of 0.89 which is also not significant (p = 0.0646) but is directionally consistent with an inverse relationship. The gradual reduction of the hazard ratios in this analysis is meaningful. In fact, when the continuous version of years of playing experience is substituted for the categorical variable, number of career years played emerges as a significant inverse predictor of mortality risk (p = 0.004, data not shown). In other words, as playing experience increases among former Major League Baseball players, mortality risk decreases.

8.7.3 Does Total Years of Playing Experience Affect the Relationship Between Race/Hispanic Origin and Mortality Risk?

See Table 8.9. Adding race/Hispanic origin to the Cox regression described in the paragraph above does not change anything with respect to the main study hypotheses. That is, controlling for year of birth and years of Major League Baseball playing experience, compared to non-Hispanic whites, there continues to be about a 40% increased risk of mortality among African-American players (p < 0.0001), as well as a 20% increased risk among Hispanic players (p = 0.0415). When continuous years of playing experience is substituted for the categorical variable, there is virtually no change in these results (data not shown). The hazard ratio for continuous years of experience is less than unity (0.986) and is significant (p = 0.0024), indicating an inverse relationship with mortality risk.

Table 8.8 Cox proportional hazards regression predicting mortality risk based on total number of Major League Baseball years played controlling for year of birth

Variables	Hazard ratio	p-value
Year of birth (continuous)	0.98	<0.0001
Total years played		
1–2 years	Index reference	
3–5 years	0.97	0.6534
6–9 years	0.98	0.753
10–14 years	0.89	0.0646
15+ years	0.81	0.0193

Table 8.9 Cox proportional hazards regression predicting mortality risk based on total number of Major League Baseball years played and race/Hispanic origin controlling for year of birth

Variables	Hazard ratio	p-value
Year of birth (continuous)	0.98	<0.0001
Total years played		
1–2 years	Index reference	
3–5 years	0.97	0.6409
6–9 years	0.98	0.6931
10–14 years	0.89	0.0721
15+ years	0.79	0.0108
Race/Hispanic origin		
African-American	1.4	<0.0001
Hispanic	1.2	0.0415
Non-Hispanic white	Index reference	

8.7.4 Summary of Empirical Results

- Total years of Major League Baseball playing experience and mortality risk are inversely related.
- Both race/Hispanic origin and total years of Major League Baseball playing experience are independent predictors of mortality.

Years of playing experience adds significantly to the prediction of mortality risk, above and beyond what is explained by year of birth and race/Hispanic origin. Unlike BMI, however, which is directly related to mortality risk, years of playing experience is an inverse predictor. Nevertheless, non-Hispanic whites have a significantly diminished risk of mortality relative to the other 2 groups when number of career years played is controlled. Like previous research in this area, length of playing career shows no sign of increasing mortality risk. Total years of playing experience will be used in the multivariate analyses in Chap. 9.

8.8 Player Position

8.8.1 Background

There is considerable evidence indicating that player position in Major League Baseball as well as other professional sports varies by race/Hispanic origin (Phillips 1983; Society for American Baseball Research no date; Schneider and Eitzen, 1986; Nightengale 2016). During the period covered by the current study, for example, there is literature indicating that Hispanics were more likely to play infield positions, African-Americans more frequently played outfield positions, and non-Hispanic whites dominated the pitching position (Society for American Baseball Research no date). Pitching especially, has been a position infrequently played by African-Americans in Major League Baseball. As recently as 2016, there were only 14 African-American pitchers on opening-day Major League Baseball rosters representing just over 3% of all pitchers in the League (Nightengale 2016). In professional football, an analogous under-representation of African-Americans at the quarterback position has been documented (Schneider and Eitzen 1986). Unevenness in the racial composition of other NFL positions, like non-Hispanic whites playing the offensive line and African-Americans playing safeties, has similarly been demonstrated (Schneider and Eitzen 1986).

Some of the imbalanced allocation of players at certain positions can be attributed to body size. However, there is also evidence that stereo-typing and prejudice play a role in this relationship. The unfortunate and fallacious stereotype that may limit African-American play in some professional sport positions relates to their being ill-equipped to master complex decision-making as well as leadership demands encom-passed by select critical positions (Edwards 1969; Nightengale 2016). This type of stereotyping, known as "centrality," increased between 1960 and 1980 (Phillips 1983), overlapping with the timeframe of the current study.

Research regarding position as a risk factor for mortality among former Major League Baseball players has been under-studied and no real relationships have been reported in the literature. However, several previous mortality studies of former base-ball players have omitted pitchers from their research (Saint Onge et al. 2008; Halpern and Coren 1991). Since pitchers typically comprise about 45% of all professional baseball players, this omission has reduced the scope and breath of several research efforts in this area.

In some sports like football, player position and body size are strongly linked. This makes it important to tease apart the role of BMI versus player position in mortality studies. For example, in the NFL, both offensive and defensive linemen have mean BMIs that are in the obese range and is significantly higher than other position categories like running backs, receivers or kickers (Markowitz 2018). In analyses of NFL players that are *not* controlled for BMI, offensive and defensive linemen have significantly elevated mortality risk. Once BMI and other important variables are controlled, however, these position types are no longer risk factors for mortality. Clearly, the study of position and mortality is a complicated one based on possible relationships with race/Hispanic origin as well as BMI.

8.9   Empirical Results

8.9.1   Player Position and Race/Hispanic Origin

8.9.1.1   2-Way Position

As can be seen in the top part of Table 8.10, there are significant differences among the 3 race/Hispanic origin groups with respect to the 2-way player position variable. More than half of all non-Hispanic white players are pitchers compared to 33% of Hispanics and only 15.7% of African-Americans ($p < 0.0001$).

8.9.1.2   5-Way Position

See the bottom part of Table 8.10. In addition to the differences in the percentage of players who are pitchers, there are differences among the 3 race/Hispanic origin groups with respect to catchers, infielders and outfielders. There is a higher percentage of non-Hispanic whites who are catchers (9.7%) compared to Hispanics (6.5%) and African-Americans (3.6%). Hispanics have the highest percentage of infielders (32.8%) compared to the other 2 groups of players who average about 20–22%. Finally, there is a much higher percentage of African-American players at the outfield position (45%) compared to Hispanics (18.4%) and non-Hispanic whites (12.5%). The overall test of race/Hispanic origin by the 5-group player position variable is significant ($p < 0.0001$).

Table 8.10   Player position by race/Hispanic origin

Player position	Race/Hispanic origin						
	African-American		Hispanic		Non-Hispanic white		
	N	%	N	%	N	%	p-value*
2-way							
Non-pitcher	495	84.3	280	67.0	2089	49.1	<0.0001
Pitcher	92	15.7	138	33.0	2169	50.9	
5-way							
Catcher	21	3.6	27	6.5	414	9.7	<0.0001
Infielder	128	21.8	137	32.8	845	19.8	
Other	82	14.0	39	9.3	300	7.1	
Outfielder	264	45.0	77	18.4	530	12.5	
Pitcher	92	15.7	138	33.0	2169	50.9	

*Based on 3×2 and 5×2 chi-square tests respectively

8.9.2 Player Position and Mortality Risk

Table 8.11 provides hazard ratio results for the 2- and 5-way player position variables predicting mortality risk controlling for year of birth. Using non-pitchers as the index reference group for the 2-way analysis, being a pitcher is associated with a significantly elevated hazard ratio of 1.14 (p = 0.0031). In the 5-way player position model that utilizes infielders as the reference group, pitchers again emerge at significant mortality risk with a hazard ratio of 1.21 (p = 0.0016).

8.9.3 Does Player Position Affect the Relationship Between Race/Hispanic Origin and Mortality Risk?

See Table 8.12. Adding race/Hispanic origin to either the 2- or 5-way position Cox regressions described in the paragraph above does not alter the relationship between race/Hispanic origin and mortality. In the 5-way position analysis, African-American as well as Hispanic players continue to be at significantly elevated risk of mortality relative to non-Hispanic white players with hazard ratios of 1.47 (p < 0.0001) and 1.23 respectively (p = 0.0244). In addition, playing the pitcher position persists as a significant independent predictor of mortality risk with a hazard ratio of 1.23 (p = 0.0005) when race/Hispanic origin is added to the analysis.

Table 8.11 Cox proportional hazards regressions predicting mortality risk based on player position controlling for year of birth

Variables	Hazard ratio	p-value
Year of birth (continuous)	0.98	<0.0001
Player position		
2-way		
Non-pitcher	Index reference	
Pitcher	1.14	0.0031
5-way		
Catcher	1.15	0.1118
Infielder	Index reference	
Other	1.12	0.2292
Outfielder	1.05	0.5003
Pitcher	1.21	0.0016

Table 8.12 Cox proportional
hazards regressions
predicting mortality risk
based on player position and
race/Hispanic origin
controlling for year of birth

Variables	Hazard ratio	p-value
Year of birth (continuous)	0.97	<0.0001
Player position		
2-way		
Non-pitcher	Index reference	
Pitcher	1.18	0.0004
Race/Hispanic origin		
African-American	1.45	<0.0001
Hispanic	1.22	0.0293
Non-Hispanic white	Index reference	
5-way		
Infielder	Index reference	
Catcher	1.17	0.07
Other	1.11	0.2861
Outfielder	1.01	0.8888
Pitcher	1.23	0.0005
Race/Hispanic origin		
African-American	1.47	<0.0001
Hispanic	1.23	0.0244
Non-Hispanic white	Index reference	

8.9.4   Summary of Empirical Results

- There are significant differences among the 3 race/Hispanic origin groups with respect to player position. There are significantly more non-Hispanic white pitchers, more African-American outfielders, and more Hispanic infielders.
- Controlling for year of birth only, pitchers are at elevated risk of mortality.
- When race is added to the analysis, playing the pitcher position continues to be a significant independent risk factor for mortality.
- African-American as well as Hispanic players persist at a mortality disadvantage relative to non-Hispanic whites when year of birth and player position are included in the analysis.

The results provided in this chapter confirm the established fact that player position in Major League Baseball is intertwined with race/Hispanic origin. The under-representation of African-Americans as pitchers, a practice that cannot be fully explained by body size, is one of the key elements of this unevenness. Player position is also statistically related to mortality risk with pitchers having a disadvantage. Nevertheless, when year of birth and position are controlled in the analyses, race/Hispanic origin persists as a risk factor for mortality. These results justify the inclusion of player position in more definitive multivariate analyses that will be undertaken in Chap. 9. It will be important to determine whether the elevated risk of pitchers is related to other significant mortality predictors, particularly BMI.

8.10 Handedness

8.10.1 Background

About 90% of humans are right-handed (McManus 2009). Because there appears to be certain advantages to being left-handed in baseball, both offensively and defensively, the percentage of lefties is higher among Major League Baseball players compared to the general population (Peterson 2017). This avails opportunities to study handedness and mortality in cohorts of baseball players.

There have been several published studies that point to the possibility of mortality advantages among right-handers in the general population. One author goes so far as to say that "…the literature now contains hundreds of studies that show that left-handedness is associated with a wide range of health-risk factors including serious accidents, immune system disorders, and birth-related complications …." (Coren and Halpern 1993). Yet, no empirical data are presented in this paper to support the authors' contention that "… left-handedness is a marker for reduced longevity" (Coren and Halpern 1993).

Several papers have appeared in the scientific literature that indicate that left-handed athletes are at increased risk of accident-related injuries as well as deaths from unnatural causes (Aggleton et al. 1993, 1994; Halpern and Coren 1991). One study indicates that the average age at death is 9 years younger for left-handed individuals (Halpern and Coren 1991). Based on this difference, the questionable conclusion is reached that lefties have higher mortality rates. However, death rates and age at death are different measures since the underlying populations compared may have disparate year of birth distributions that impact on their age at death. In fact, many studies on handedness find no increased mortality among lefties compared to righties (Salive et al. 1993; Wolf et al. 1991; Kuhlmeier 1991).

There has also been some Major League Baseball mortality research that has examined the influence of handedness. One study yielded a p-value of 0.13 in the direction of a mortality advantages for righties (Abel and Kruger 2004). While interesting, however, significant associations for a relationship between handedness and mortality have not been uncovered among Major League Baseball players (Panjer 1993; Saint Onge et al. 2008).

In brief, there is some limited, but mixed and contentious evidence from both general population and professional athlete studies regarding health advantages, and possibly lower mortality risk for righties compared to lefties. Because of this and given the availability of handedness data for players in the current study cohort, it seems worthy of examination here.

8.11   Empirical Results

8.11.1   Handedness and Race/Hispanic Origin

8.11.1.1   Batting

See the top part of Table 8.13 for a cross-tabulation of race/Hispanic origin by hand-edness which indicates that there are significant differences among the 3 groups of players (p < 0.0001). Hispanics are less likely to bat from the left side of home plate (15.1%) and more likely to bat from the right side (76.6%) than their African-American (32.5% lefty batters and 52.6% righty) and non-Hispanic white counter-parts (28.7% lefty batters and 66% righty).

8.11.1.2   Throwing

The bottom half of Table 8.13 provides the results for throwing handedness and again, there are significant differences among the 3 race/Hispanic origin groups (p = 0.0004). A higher percentage of Hispanic players (85.9%) throw with their right hands compared to African-Americans (80.8%) and non-Hispanic whites (78%).

8.11.2   Handedness and Mortality Risk

Analyses that control for year of birth and assess the role of handedness on mortality risk are shown in Table 8.14. These results indicate that neither batting nor throwing handedness is associated with mortality risk.

Table 8.13   Handedness by race/Hispanic origin

Handedness	Race/Hispanic origin						
	African-American		Hispanic		Non-Hispanic white		p-value*
	N	%	N	%	N	%	
Batting							
Both	87	14.8	35	8.4	228	5.4	<0.0001
Left	191	32.5	63	15.1	1221	28.7	
Right	309	52.6	320	76.6	2809	66.0	
Throwing							
Left	113	19.3	59	14.1	937	22.0	0.0004
Right	474	80.8	359	85.9	3321	78.0	

*Based on 3 × 3 and 3 × 2 chi-square tests respectively

Table 8.14 Cox proportional hazards regressions predicting mortality risk based on handedness controlling for year of birth

Variables	Hazard ratio	p-value
Year of birth (continuous)	0.98	<0.0001
Handedness		
Batting		
Right	Index reference	
Left	0.98	0.6117
Both	0.85	0.1392
Throwing		
Right	Index reference	
Left	0.97	0.5618

8.11.3 Does Handedness Affect the Relationship Between Race/Hispanic Origin and Mortality Risk?

Because handedness is completely unrelated to mortality risk, there is no need to analyze it further. Additionally, handedness will not be included in the multivariate analyses.

8.11.4 Summary of Empirical Results

- There are significant differences among the 3 race/Hispanic origin groups with respect to handedness. There are more Hispanics who throw and bat right
- There are significant differences among the 3 race/Hispanic origin groups with respect to handedness. There are more Hispanics who throw and bat right.
- There is no relationship between throwing or batting handedness and mortality risk.

Existing studies purporting a link between handedness and mortality must be considered with caution since false conclusions are possible. While handedness is statistically related to race/Hispanic origin, it has no effect on mortality among former Major League Baseball players.

References

Abel, E. L., & Kruger, M. L. (2004). Left-handed major-league baseball players and longevity re-examined. *Perceptual and Motor Skills, 99*(3), 990–992.

Abel, E. L., & Kruger, M. L. (2005). The longevity of baseball Hall of Famers compared to other players. *Death Studies, 29,* 959–963.

Aggleton, J. P., Kentridge, R. W., & Neaw, N. (1993). Evidence for longevity differences between left handed and right handed men. *Journal of Epidemiology and Community Health, 47,* 206–209.

Aggleton, J. P., Bland, J. M., Kentridge, R. W., & Neave, N. J. (1994). Handedness and longevity. *British Medical Journal, 309,* 1681–1684.

Allison, D. B., Fontaine, K. R., Manson, J. E., Stevens, J., & Vanitalie, T. B. (1999). Annual deaths attributable to obesity in the United States. *JAMA, 282,* 1530–1538.

Badenhausen, K. (2016). Average baseball salary up 20,700% since first CBA in 1968. *Forbes*, April 7. Retrieved from https://www.forbes.com/sites/kurtbadenhausen/2016/04/07/average-baseball-salary-up-20700-since-first-cba-in-1968/#2af2946a3e48.

Baron, S. L., & Rinsky, R. (1994). *Health hazard evaluation report, National Football League players mortality study.* Report No. HETA 88-085. Atlanta: Centers for Disease Control and Prevention/National Institute for Occupational Safety and Health. Retrieved from https://www.cdc.gov/niosh/hhe/reports/pdfs/1988-0085-letter.pdf?id=10.26616/NIOSHHETA88085.

Baron, S. L., Heim, M. J., Lehman, E., & Gersic, C. M. (2012). Body mass index, playing position, race, and the cardiovascular mortality of retired professional football players. *American Journal of Cardiology, 109,* 889–896.

Berrington de Gonzalez, A., Hartge, P., Cerhan, J. R., Flint, J. R., Hannan, L., MacInnis, R. J., et al. (2010). Body-mass index and mortality among 1.46 million white adults. *New England Journal of Medicine, 363,* 2211–2219.

CDC (2018). *United States Cancer Statistics (USCS).* Retrieved from https://www.cdc.gov/cancer/npcr/uscs/index.htm.

CDC, Centers for Disease Control and Prevention (2015). *About adult BMI.* Retrieved from https://www.cdc.gov/healthyweight/assessing/bmi/adult_bmi/.

Clarke, P., O'Malley, P. M., Johnston, L. D., & Schulenberg, J. E. (2009). Social disparities in BMI trajectories across adulthood by gender, race/ethnicity and lifetime socio-economic position: 1986–2004. *International Journal of Epidemiology, 38*(2), 499–509.

Coren, S., & Halpern, D. F. (1993). A replay of the baseball data. *Perceptual and Motor Skills, 76*(2), 403–406.

Deurenberg-Yap, M., & Deurenberg, P. (2003). Is a re-evaluation of WHO body mass index cut-off values needed? *Nutrition Reviews, 61,* S80–S87.

Diehr, P., Koepsell, T., Cheadle, A., Psaty, B. M., Wagner, E., & Curry, S. (1993). Do communities differ in health behaviors? *Journal of Clinical Epidemiology, 46,* 1141–1149.

Diez Roux, A. V. (2001). Investigating neighborhood and area effects on health. *American Journal of Public Health, 91*(11), 1783–1789.

Edwards, H. (1969). *The revolt of the Black athlete.* New York: Free Press.

Flegal, K. M., Carroll, M., Ogden, C. L., & Johnson, C. L. (2002). Prevalence and trends in obesity among US adults, 1999–2000. *JAMA, 288,* 1723–1727.

Flegal, K. M., Graubard, B. I., Williamson, D. F., & Gail, M. H. (2007). Cause-specific excess deaths associated with underweight, overweight, and obesity. *JAMA, 298,* 2028–2037.

GBD 2015 Obesity Collaborators (2017). Health effects of overweight and obesity in 195 countries over 25 years. *New England Journal of Medicine, 377,* 13–27.

Govil, S. R., Weidner, G., Merritt-Worden, T., & Ornish, D. (2009). Socioeconomic status and improvements in lifestyle, coronary risk factors, and quality of life. *American Journal of Public Health, 99*(7), 1263–1270.

Hales, C. M., Carroll, M. D., Fryar, C. D., & Ogden, C. L. (2017). Prevalence of obesity among adults and youth: United States, 2015–2016. *NCHS Data Brief, 288,* 1–8.

Halpern, D. F., & Coren, S. (1991). Handedness and life span. *New England Journal of Medicine, 324,* 998. Letter.

Hojjat, T. A., & Hojatt, R. (2017). *The economics of obesity.* Singapore: Springer.

Hsu, W. C., Boyko, E. J., Fujimoto, W. Y., Kanaya, A., Karmally, W., Karter, A., et al. (2012). Pathophysiologic differences among Asians, native Hawaiians, and other Pacific Islanders and treatment implications. *Diabetes Care, 35,* 1189–1198.

Kassirer, J. P., & Angell, M. (1998). Losing weight—An ill-fated New Year's resolution. *New England Journal of Medicine, 338,* 52–54.

Kuhlmeier, K. V. (1991). Longevity and left-handedness. *American Journal of Public Health, 81,* 513. Letter.

Lawler, T., Lawler, F., Gibson, J., & Murray, R. (2012). Does the African-American-white mortality gap persist after playing professional basketball? A 50-year historical cohort study. *Annals of Epidemiology, 22,* 406–412.

Markowitz, J. S. (2018). *Mortality and its risk factors among professional athletes: A comparison between former NBA and NFL players.* Cham: Springer.

McManus, I. (2009). The history and geography of human handedness. In I. Sommer & R. Kahn (Eds.), *Language lateralization and psychosis.* UK: Cambridge University Press. Retrieved from https://www.ucl.ac.uk/medical-education/publications/reprints2009/2009-History_GeographyOfHumanHandedness.pdf.

Mitchell, N., Catenacci, V., Wyatt, H. R., & Hill, J. O. (2011). Obesity: Overview of an epidemic. *Psychiatric Clinics of North America, 34*(4), 717–732.

Nightengale, B. (2016). As MLB celebrates Jackie Robinson, dearth of black pitchers concerns many. *USA Today.* Retrieved from https://www.usatoday.com/story/sports/columnist/bob-nightengale/2016/04/14/mlb-jackie-robinson-african-american-players-pitchers/83052454/.

Nuttall, F. Q. (2015). Body mass index: Obesity, BMI, and health: A critical review. *Nutrition Today, 50*(3), 117–128.

Panjer, H. H. (1993). 1994-01 mortality differences by handedness. *Transactions of Society of Actuaries, 45,* 257–274.

Peterson, D. (2017). *Righties vs lefties—The importance of handedness training in baseball hitting.* Retrieved from http://www.gamesensesports.com/knowledge/2017/3/17/righties-vs-lefties-the-importance-of-handedness-training-in-baseball-hitting.

Phillips, J. C. (1983). Race and career opportunities in Major League Baseball: 1960–1980. *Journal of Sport and Social Issues, 7*(2), 1–17.

Prospective Studies Collaboration. (2009). Body-mass index and cause-specific mortality in 900,000 adults. *Lancet, 373,* 1083–1096.

SABR, Society for American Baseball Research (no date). *Baseball demographics, 1947–2016.* Retrieved from https://sabr.org/bioproj/topic/baseball-demographics-1947-2012.

Saint Onge, J. M., Rogers, R. G., & Kruger, P. M. (2008). Major League Baseball players' life expectancies. *Social Science Quarterly, 89*(3), 817–830.

Salive, M. E., Guralnik, J. M., & Glynn, R. J. (1993). Left-handedness and mortality. *American Journal of Public Health, 83*(2), 265–267.

Schneider, J. J., & Eitzen, D. S. (1986). Racial segregation by professional football positions. *Social Science Research, 70*(4), 259–261.

Scully, G. (1973). Economic discrimination in professional sports. *Law and Contemporary Problems, 38*(1), 67–84.

Seo, D. C., & Torabi, M. R. (2006). Racial/ethnic differences in body mass index, morbidity and Attitudes toward obesity among U.S. adults. *Journal of National Medical Associations, 98*(8), 1300–1308.

Shaikin, B. (2016). A look at how Major League Baseball salaries have grown more than 20,000% the last 50 years. *Los Angeles Times.* Retrieved from https://www.latimes.com/sports/mlb/la-sp-mlb-salaries-chart-20160329-story.html.

Social Security Administration. (2015). *National average wage index.* Retrieved from https://www.ssa.gov/oact/cola/AWI.html.

US Census Bureau (no date). *Explore Census Data.* Retrieved from https://data.census.gov/cedsci/landing?intcmp=data_cedsci_banner.html.

Wagner, D. R., & Heyward, V. H. (2000). Measures of body composition in blacks and whites. *American Journal of Clinical Nutrition, 71,* 1392–1402.

W.H.O. Fact Sheet (2016). *Obesity and overweight.* Retrieved from http://www.who.int/mediacentre/factsheets/fs311/en/.

W.H.O. (2017). *World health statistics, 2017*. Retrieved from http://www.who.int/gho/publications/world_health_statistics/2017/en/.

Wolf, P. A., D'Agostino, R. B., & Cobb, J. (1991). Left-handedness and life expectancy. *New England Journal of Medicine, 325*, 1042. Letter.

Yen, I., & Kaplan, G. (1999). Neighborhood social environment and risk of death. *American Journal of Epidemiology, 149*, 898–907.

Yen, I., & Syme, S. L. (1999). The social environment and health. *Annual Review of Public Health, 20*, 287–308.

Chapter 9
Final Multivariate Testing of Study Hypotheses

9.1 Methods

All analyses in this chapter will exclude birthplace region and handedness for reasons already explained.

The first analysis in this chapter predicting mortality risk includes *all categories* of all significant study variables, i.e., race/Hispanic origin, year of birth, educational attainment, BMI, pitcher position, and years of playing experience. Using stepwise backwards elimination methods with all-cause mortality as the dependent variable, non-significant items will be removed from the model one at a time until only significant items remain. The order of variable removal will be based on p-values with the highest p-values removed first. Year of birth, BMI and total years of Major League Baseball playing experience are continuous variables. A final multivariate model will substitute the continuous versions of these variables for their categorical counterparts.

9.2 Empirical Results

9.2.1 Multivariate Analysis Using Categorical Variables

All significant study variables are initially entered simultaneously as categorical items into a stepwise backwards elimination multivariate Cox proportional hazards regression predicting mortality risk. These results are shown on the left side of Table 9.1. Of note, none of the years of Major League Baseball playing experience categories are significant in this model and, consequently, this variable is dropped from the analysis. As shown on the right side of Table 9.1, all other remaining variables are significant independent predictors of mortality risk. Consequently, this is deemed the final multivariate model using categorical variables. The results of this analysis indicate that African-American players have a 41% increased risk of mortality relative to non-Hispanic whites which is significant ($p < 0.0001$). The hazard ratio for Hispanics is 1.01 and is not statistically significant ($p = 0.8993$) compared to non-Hispanic whites. These results are very similar to the ones shown previously in Chap. 7 when the inclusion of educational attainment in the analysis diminished mortality risk differences between Hispanics and non-Hispanic whites.

See the right side of Table 9.1 for the results of the second step of the backwards elimination multivariate analysis that uses categorical variables with years of playing experience eliminated. Using 1955–1966 as the index reference, each older year of birth category yields progressively higher hazard ratios that are all significant. For example, players born between 1945 and 1954 have a hazard ratio of 1.71 ($p = 0.0021$) and players born the earliest, i.e., 1905–1914, have a hazard ratio of 3.3 ($p < 0.0001$). In other words, and as expected, year of birth categories and mortality risk are inversely related. The results for educational attainment also indicate an inverse relationship; as education level increases, mortality risk decreases. Using players with the highest educational attainment as the index group, i.e., 3 or more years of college completed, hazard ratios rise with each lower level of educational attainment. For example, players with little or no high school have a hazard ratio of 1.58 ($p < 0.0001$) and those with some high school have a hazard ratio of 1.35 ($p = 0.0002$). Compared to players with normal BMIs, individuals who are overweight are at significant mortality risk (hazard ratio $= 1.19$; $p = 0.0002$) in this same multivariate analysis. Using the 5-way player position variable with infielders as the index group, pitchers continue to be at significant risk of mortality (hazard ratio $= 1.18$; $p = 0.0055$). Since all variables are significant in this second step, this becomes the final multivariate (categorical) model.

9.2.2 *Multivariate Analysis Using Continuous Variables*

See Table 9.2. In a second Cox proportional hazards regression predicting mortality risk with all significant variables included, year of birth, BMI, and years of Major League Baseball playing experience are entered as continuous variables. Race/Hispanic origin and educational attainment continue to be used as categorical variables in this analysis. While the categorical version of playing experience fails to be significant, there is a significant inverse relationship when this item is included as a continuous variable (hazard ratio $= 0.99$; $p = 0.0119$). Because all the variables predicting mortality risk are significant in this first step, no variables are dropped from this analysis and this is declared the final (continuous) multivariate model. Compared to non-Hispanic white players, African-Americans continue to be at elevated risk with a hazard ratio of 1.43 ($p < 0.0001$), and Hispanic origin is *not* significant (hazard ratio=1.04; $p = 0.6673$). Year of birth (hazard ratio $= 0.99$; $p < 0.0001$) and BMI (hazard ratio $= 1.06$; $p = 0.0004$) continue to be significant as continuous variables. The other hazard ratios for the categorical variables, i.e., educational attainment and pitcher position, remain significant independent predictors of mortality risk and resemble the hazard ratios described in the previous paragraph.

Table 9.1 Stepwise backwards elimination Cox proportional hazards regression predicting mortality risk using categorical variables

Variables (categorical)	First step; all variables entered[a]		Second step; eliminate years of playing experience	
	Hazard ratio	p-value	Hazard ratio	p-value
Race/Hispanic origin				
African-American	1.42	<0.0001	1.41	<0.0001
Hispanic	1.02	0.839	1.01	0.8993
Non-Hispanic white	Index reference		Index reference	
Year of birth				
1905–1914	3.38	<0.0001	3.3	<0.0001
1915–1924	3.13	<0.0001	3.14	<0.0001
1925–1934	2.57	<0.0001	2.59	<0.0001
1935–1944	2.0	<0.0001	2.01	<0.0001
1945–1954	1.71	0.0021	1.71	0.0021
1955–1966	Index reference		Index reference	
Educational attainment				
Little or no high school	1.57	<0.0001	1.58	<0.0001
At least some high school, but no college	1.37	0.0001	1.5	0.0002
Some college, but unknown number of years completed	1.17	0.0842	1.17	0.0866
1–2 years of college completed	1.11	0.2676	1.1	0.2899
3 or more years of college completed	Index reference		Index reference	
BMI				
Normal	Index reference		Index reference	
Overweight	1.19	0.0002	1.19	0.0002
Total years played Major League Baseball				
1–2 year	Index		Eliminated	
3–5 year	0.98	0.719		
6–9 year	1.0	0.98		
10–14 years	0.95	0.4237		
15+ years	0.85	0.0799		
5-way position				
Infielder	Index reference		Index reference	
Catcher	1.08	0.3848	1.09	0.3499
Other	1.01	0.9533	1.03	0.7569
Outfielder	0.98	0.8011	0.98	0.7506
Pitcher	1.17	0.008	1.18	0.0055

[a]Birthplace region and handedness have been excluded from these analyses

Table 9.2 Stepwise backwards elimination multivariate Cox proportional hazards regression predicting mortality risk using continuous variables

Variables	First and final step[a]	
	Hazard ratio	p-value*
Race/Hispanic origin		
African-American	1.43	<0.0001
Hispanic	1.04	0.6673
Non-Hispanic white	Index reference	
Year of birth (continuous)	0.98	<0.0001
Educational attainment		
Little or no high school	1.56	<0.0001
At least some high school, but no college	1.39	<0.0001
Some college, but unknown number of years completed	1.19	0.0519
1–2 years of college completed	1.13	0.196
3 or more years of college completed	Index reference	
BMI (continuous)	1.06	0.0004
Total years played Major League Baseball (continuous)	0.99	0.0119
5-way position		
Infielder	Index reference	
Catcher	1.07	0.4804
Other	1.01	0.9505
Outfielder	0.99	0.8684
Pitcher	1.16	0.0112

*Birthplace region and handedness have been excluded from these analyses

[a] All variables entered are significant making this the final model

9.3   Post hoc Analysis of Mortality Risk Between Hispanic and Non-Hispanic White Players Stratified by Education

Analyses presented in Chap. 7 indicate that when educational attainment, year of birth, and race/Hispanic are included in a Cox regression, mortality risk is *not* elevated among Hispanic origin players relative to non-Hispanic whites. This result is quite different from the one reported in Chap. 6 which shows significant mortality risk among Hispanic players compared to non-Hispanic whites when educational attainment is omitted from the analysis. The results presented in Chap. 7 lead to the preliminary conclusion that educational attainment is mediating the role of Hispanic origin on mortality to the point where mortality risk is similar between Hispanic and non-Hispanic white players. Such a finding would be consistent with the presence of a Hispanic Paradox. The multivariate results presented in this chapter that simultaneously control for all other significant variables provide further support for this conclusion.

To examine this further, a post hoc analysis stratified by educational attainment will be attempted to help clarify whether mortality risk is similar or different between Hispanic and non-Hispanic white players. However, there are too few Hispanic players with any college education (n = 16) to conduct a completely stratified analysis. As an alternative, a Cox regression that controls for all the significant variables is conducted *within* Hispanic (n = 402) and non-Hispanic players (n = 1851) who completed less than a college education. With non-Hispanic whites as the index reference, the hazard ratio is 1.08 reflecting a small (8%) increased mortality risk for Hispanics that is not significant (p = 0.4286, data not shown). These post hoc results provide some additional evidence that the mortality risk between Hispanic and non-Hispanic white players is similar—at least within players with no college education.

9.3.1   Summary of Empirical Results

- There continues to be support for the hypothesis that compared to non-Hispanic white players, and considering all other significant study variables simultaneously, African-American race is a significant independent risk factor for mortality.
- Hispanic origin, a significant predictor of mortality in analyses that do not contain educational attainment, fails to be significant compared to non-Hispanic white players when education is included.
- In addition to African-American race, more distal year of birth, lower educational attainment, higher BMI, and playing the pitcher position remain significant predictors of mortality risk in these more definitive analyses.
- While year of birth, BMI, playing the pitcher position are independent risk factors for mortality, they do not influence the relationship between race/Hispanic and mortality.
- There is a significant inverse relationship between (continuous) years of experience and mortality risk. While not significant, the results for the years of playing experience categories show a similar trend.
- Post hoc analysis within players with less than a college education indicates that mortality risk between Hispanic and non-Hispanic white players is similar. This result provides some additional support to the possibility of there being a Hispanic Paradox in the study cohort.

Considering all the significant variables in this study simultaneously, compared to non-Hispanic whites, African-American players have significantly elevated mortality risk. The mortality risk of Hispanic players is more complicated since it is influenced by educational attainment. Adding to this complexity is the vastly uneven distributions of educational attainment for the 3 study groups. Hispanic players are so poorly educated relative to non-Hispanic whites and African-Americans that the findings related to educational attainment must be cautiously interpreted. Additional discussion on this will follow in Chap. 11.

Part IV
External Analysis and Discussion

Chapter 10
Comparison of Mortality Rates Between Major League Baseball Players and the General Population

10.1 Background

All the previous analyses contained in this book can be considered "internal" since they are conducted within groups of former Major League Baseball players in the study cohort. This logically follows from the internal nature of the study hypotheses. Attention is now turned to "external" analyses of mortality rates between the players and the US general population. The research question for these external analyses is whether mortality rates of former Major League Baseball players is higher, lower, or about the same as rates in the US population. To be most meaningful, this question will be asked within the 3 race/Hispanic origin groups. The results of this external analyses provide additional clues and context for understanding and interpreting the internal study results.

Just like NBA and NFL players, former Major League Baseball players should be considered "elite athletes." Like Olympians and other international athletes that compete at a world-class level, professional baseball players are the best in the world at what they do. Strength, speed, agility and other forms of athleticism are common among Major League Baseball players. For many elite athletes, reaching the pinnacle of their respective sports represents a lifetime of dedication and hard-work.

There is a considerable scientific literature documenting mortality advantages for a wide range of elite athletes. On an international level, the list of athletes that have been shown to have superior mortality outcomes compared to a range of general population and other control groups include Finnish male endurance athletes (Sarna et al. 1997), team and power sports athletes (Kettunen et al. 2014), professional divers from Norway (Irgens et al. 2013), male Olympic team athletes from Poland (Poznańska and Gajewski 2001), French elite road cyclists (Morcet et al. 2012) athletes from 9 different countries who have won Olympic medals (Clarke et al. 2012), and endurance cross-country skiers (Grimsmo et al. 2011). Finally, in a review of 57 articles addressing this topic, 54 of which were peer-reviewed, there are only 2 studies that fail to uncover mortality advantages among athletes when compared to

© The Author(s), under exclusive license to Springer Nature Switzerland AG 2019
J. S. Markowitz, *Mortality Among Hispanic and African-American Players After Desegregation in Major League Baseball*, SpringerBriefs in Public Health,
https://doi.org/10.1007/978-3-030-17280-0_10

age- and gender- matched controls from the general population (Lemez and Baker 2015).

Mortality outcomes among former athletes who played professional US sports are also consistently better than ones obtained from otherwise comparable US general populations. This includes several studies of former Major League Baseball players who played during varying periods of time (Saint Onge et al. 2008; Abel and Kruger 2006; Waterbor et al. 1988; MetLife 1975). Abel and Kruger (2006), for example, found that Major League Baseball players who debuted between 1900 and 1939 had a life expectancy that was nearly 5 years longer than an age-adjusted control group of males drawn from the general population. A similar life expectancy advantage for Major League Baseball players who debuted as players over a 102-year period, from 1902 to 2004, was demonstrated by Saint Onge and colleagues (2008).

Compared to general populations that have been selected using a range of method-ologies, mortality advantages among groups of professional basketball and football players have also been documented. For example, Lawler and colleagues (2012) report a 5-year life expectancy advantage for a large sample of professional bas-ketball players who played anytime between 1946 and 2005 when compared to race-stratified males from the US general population. Similarly, Markowitz (2018) obtained significant SMRs for comparisons between a cohort of NBA players who played in the league anytime between 1960 and 1986 and the general population. The overall SMR for African-American and white NBA players versus their age- and race-matched general population controls is 0.48 and 0.56 respectively, again depicting lower mortality rates for the athletes (Markowitz 2018).

While surprising to some readers, mortality advantages have also been consistently uncovered among former NFL players compared to the US general population. Both NIOSH studies published in 1994 with a relatively young cohort of former NFL players averaging just over 40 years of age (Baron and Rinsky 1994), as well as a 17-year follow-up study of many of these same players (Baron et al. 2012; Lehman et al. 2012) provide significantly more favorable all-cause mortality results for African-American and white players compared to general populations of males. Overall SMRs for players in the 2 race groups average about 0.5 reflecting a 50% decrease in mortality rates among NFL players relative to males from the general population (Baron et al. 2012; Lehman et al. 2012). Similar SMR results have also been obtained by Markowitz (2018) with respect to African-American (SMR = 0.42) and white NFL players (SMR = 0.56) versus their general population counterparts.

10.2 Methods

It is worth noting that unlike the Cox regressions used in the empirical analyses in previous chapters which compares mortality risk, SMRs compare rates. By compar-ing observed numbers of deaths among cohort members to expected values in the general population, SMRs can be generated within each race/Hispanic origin group. Expected numbers of deaths are derived from 2012 US life table data for males published in 2016 (Arias et al. 2016). Separate life tables in this CDC publication are available for whites, African-Americans and Hispanics. Of note, Hispanics in these life tables are US residents, and may not have been born in a Latin American country. This differs from Hispanic players in the current study who are all born in a Latin American country and may not have officially resided in the US.

A very large majority of Major League Baseball players, about 96%, make their professional playing debuts sometime after the age of 20 years. Consequently, players who make it to Major League Baseball are very unlikely to die before the age of 20. In fact, only 1 player in the study cohort died before the age of 20. Accordingly, a decision was made to use life table data beginning at age 20, as the use of statistics for younger ages would unduly bias the comparisons in favor of the players. Specifically, the number of observed deaths, will be calculated for each race/Hispanic origin group of players within the following 8 age strata:

- 20–29 years
- 30–39 years
- 40–49 years
- 50–59 years
- 60–69 years
- 70–79 years
- 80–99 years
- 90+ years.

SMRs are calculated for each of the 8 age strata and for each of the race/Hispanic origin groups overall. SMRs that exceed unity reflect elevated mortality rates for the players, while values below 1 indicate lower rates. For example, a hypothetical SMR of 2 reflects a mortality rate that is twice as high among players compared to controls in the US general population. An SMR of 0.7 indicates a 30% reduced rate of mortality among the players. SMR confidence intervals are provided for each age strata and for the overall SMRs. Intervals that exclude unity are statistically significant. P-values will be given for overall SMRs, i.e., all age strata combined, within each race/Hispanic origin group.

10.3 Empirical Results

The results in this chapter are divided into 3 sections, 1 for each race/Hispanic origin comparison between the Major League Baseball players and their respective counterparts in the general population.

All SMR results are shown in Table 10.1.

Table 10.1 Standardized mortality rate (SMR) results for comparisons between Major League Baseball players in 3 race/Hispanic origin groups versus their general population counterparts

Race/Hispanic origin

Age strata	African-American					Hispanic					Non-Hispanic white				
	Observed # deaths	Expected # deaths	SMR	95% normal confidence limits (SMR)		Observed # deaths	Expected # deaths	SMR	95% normal confidence limits (SMR)		Observed # deaths	Expected # deaths	SMR	95% normal confidence limits (SMR)	
				Lower bound	Upper bound				Lower bound	Upper bound				Lower bound	Upper bound
20–29	5	11.1	0.45	0.06	0.85	4	3.9	1.02	0.02	2.01	15	52.9	0.28	0.14	0.43
30–39	6	14.1	0.43	0.09	0.77	6	4.8	1.25	0.25	2.24	36	67.2	0.54	0.36	0.71
40–49	14	24.6	0.57	0.27	0.87	13	9.3	1.4	0.64	2.15	74	127.3	0.58	0.45	0.71
50–59	32	59.4	0.54	0.35	0.73	24	22.8	1.05	0.63	1.48	207	294.2	0.7	0.61	0.8
60–69	48	84.6	0.57	0.41	0.73	29	35	0.83	0.53	1.13	345	486.2	0.71	0.63	0.78
70–79	35	67.3	0.52	0.35	0.69	35	39.4	0.89	0.59	1.18	472	651.7	0.72	0.66	0.79
80–89	16	36.9	0.43	0.22	0.65	19	35.4	0.54	0.3	0.78	466	626.1	0.74	0.68	0.81
90+	2	5	0.4	0	0.95	4	4	1	0.02	1.98	111	174	0.64	0.52	0.76
All	158	303	0.52	0.44	0.6	134	154.7	0.87	0.72	1.01	1726	2479.6	0.7	0.66	0.73
p-value[a]	<0.0001					0.0744					<0.0001				

[a]Based on All

10.3.1 African-American Players Versus African-Americans in the General Population

Within all 8 age strata, the expected number of deaths in the African-American general population exceeds the observed values for African-American Major League Baseball players. Consequently, all these SMRs are less than unity; moreover, they are all statistically significant. The overall SMR for African-Americans is 0.52 and is also significant (p < 0.0001) reflecting a 48% decreased mortality rate among African-Americans players relative to their general population controls.

10.3.2 Hispanic Players Versus Hispanics in the General Population

Within Hispanics, for the 4 age strata under 60 years of age, the observed number of deaths is slightly higher than the expected values. Hence, the SMRs for these 4 age strata are slightly greater than unity indicating lower (non-significant) mortality rates among this sub-group of general population Hispanics relative to the players. Beginning with the 60–69 age stratum, the SMRs are less than 1 indicating lower death rates for the Hispanic players compared to the general population of Hispanics. The age stratum 90 years and over has an SMR of exactly 1. The overall SMR for Hispanics is 0.87 and is not significant (p = 0.0744). This means that overall death rates among Hispanic players is about 13% less than Hispanics from the general population, but this difference fails to reach significant levels.

10.3.3 Non-Hispanic White Players Versus Whites in the General Population

As is the case with African-Americans, all observed numbers of deaths for non-Hispanic white players are less than the expected values for whites in the general population. This results in SMRs less than 1 for every age stratum indicating lower death rates among players. These SMRs as well as the overall SMR for non-Hispanic whites are all significant. The overall SMR for non-Hispanic white players is 0.7 reflecting a 30% decreased mortality rate among players relative to non-Hispanic whites in the general population (p < 0.0001).

10.4   Empirical Summary

- Compared to African-Americans in the general population, African-American players have significantly lower death rates. This is the case for every age stratum and overall.
- Compared to Hispanics in the general population, the overall death rate among players is lower, although the difference is not significant.
- Compared to whites in the general population, non-Hispanic white players have significantly lower death rates. This is the case for every age stratum and overall.

Predictably, Major League Baseball players have lower mortality rates than matched controls from the general population. The results for non-Hispanic whites and African-Americans are quite robust. While not significant for Hispanic players, the directionality of their results is consistent with the 2 race groups. Possible explanations for these results will be provided in Chap. 11.

References

Abel, E. L., & Kruger, M. L. (2006). The healthy worker effect in major league baseball revisited. *Research in Sports Medicine, 14,* 83–87.

Arias, E. Heron, M., & Xu, J. (2016). United States life tables, 2012. *National Vital Statistics Report, 65*(8). Retrieved from https://www.cdc.gov/nchs/data/nvsr/nvsr65/nvsr65_08.pdf.

Baron, S., & Rinsky, R. (1994). *Health hazard evaluation report, National Football League players mortality study.* Report No. HETA 88–085. Atlanta, GA: Centers for Disease Control and Prevention, National Institute for Occupational Safety and Health. Retrieved from http://www.cdc.gov/niosh/pdfs/nflfactsheet.pdf.

Baron, S. L., Hein, M. J., Lehman, E., & Gersic, C. M. (2012). Body mass index, playing position, race, and the cardiovascular mortality of retired professional football players. *American Journal of Cardiology, 109,* 889–896.

Clarke, P. M., Walter, S. J., Hayen, A., Mallon, W. J., Heijmans, J., & Studdert, D. M. (2012). Survival of the fittest: Retrospective cohort study of the longevity of Olympic medalists in the modern era. *British Medical Journal, 345,* e8308.

Grimsmo, J., Maehlum, S., Moelstad, P., & Arnesen, H. (2011). Mortality and cardiovascular morbidity among long-term endurance male cross country skiers followed for 28–30 years. *Scandinavian Journal of Medicine and Science in Sports, 21,* 351–358.

Irgens, Å., Troland, K., Thorsen, E., & Grønning, M. (2013). Mortality among professional divers in Norway. *Occupational Medicine, 63,* 537–543.

Kettunen, J. A., Kujala, U. M., Kaprio, J., Bäckmand, H., Peltonen, M., Eriksson, J. G., & Sarna, S. (2014). All-cause and disease-specific mortality among male, former elite athletes. *British Journal of Sports Medicine, 13,* 893–897.

Lawler, T., Lawler, F., Gibson, J., & Murray, R. (2012) Does the African-American-White mortality gap persist after playing professional basketball? A 59-year historical cohort study. *Annals of Epidemiology, 22,* 406–412.

Lehman, E. J., Hein, M. J., Baron, S. L., & Gersic, C. M. (2012) Neurodegenerative causes of death among retired National Football League players. *Neurology, 79,* 1970–4.

Lemez, S., & Baker, J. (2015). Do elite athletes live longer? A systematic review of mortality and longevity in elite Athletes. *Sports Medicine Open, 1,* 16. Retrieved from https://www.ncbi.nlm.nih.gov/pmc/articles/PMC4534511/.

Markowitz, J. S. (2018). Mortality and its risk factors among professional athletes: A comparison between former NBA and NFL players. Cham: Springer Nature.

MetLife. (1975). Longevity of major league baseball players. *Statistical Bulletin of the Metropolitan Life Insurance Company, 56*, 2–4.

Morcet, J. Perrin, M. Tregaro, M., Carre, F., & Deugnier. Y. (2012). Mortality in a cohort of 514 elite road cyclists. *Science and Sports, 27*(1), 9–15.

Poznańska, A., & Gajewski, A. K. (2001). Mortality of male members of the Polish Olympic teams in 1981–1998. *Przeglad Epidemiologiczny, 55*, 305–312.

Saint Onge, J. M., Rogers, R. G., & Kruger, P. M. (2008). Major League Baseball players' life expectancies. *Social Science Quarterly, 89*(3), 817–830.

Sarna, S., Kaprio, J., Kujala, U. M., & Koskenvuo, M. (1997). Health status of former elite athletes. The finnish experience. *Aging Clinical and Experimental Research, 9*, 35–41.

Waterbor, J. C., Dezell, C. P., & Andjelkovitz, D. (1988). The mortality experience of Major League Baseball players. *New England Journal of Medicine, 318*, 1278–1280.

Chapter 11
Summary, Conclusions, and Implications

11.1 Internal Comparison Summary and Implications

The empirical analysis has demonstrated that there is a relationship between race/Hispanic origin and mortality among former Major League Baseball players. The most robust of these results pertain to race. Moreover, no variables could be identified that disrupt this association. The mortality results for Hispanic relative to non-Hispanic players are more complicated because of the impact of educational attainment.

In this book, almost all the hazard ratios derived from Cox proportional hazards models presented to this point have used non-Hispanic whites as the index reference group. Table 11.1 contains a summary of the key hazard ratios using rotating index reference groups. In other words, African-American, Hispanic and non-Hispanic white players serve as separate index reference groups for the critical between-group analyses of mortality risk. The hazard ratio results in Table 11.1 that use non-Hispanic whites as the index reference have all been shown in previous table displays. However, Table 11.1 adds the other 2 study groups as index reference groups and organizes the results into a single display that provides a comprehensive view of the key findings that will be referenced throughout this chapter.

11.1.1 African-American Versus Non-Hispanic White Mortality Comparisons

See the left side of Table 11.1. The hazard ratios between non-Hispanic white players, the index group, and African-American players range from 1.35 to 1.45 and are all statistically significant. Compared to non-Hispanic white players, African-Americans consistently have a 35–45% increased risk of mortality. While educational attainment, BMI, years of playing experience, and player position add significantly to the

© The Author(s), under exclusive license to Springer Nature Switzerland AG 2019
J. S. Markowitz, *Mortality Among Hispanic and African-American Players After Desegregation in Major League Baseball*, SpringerBriefs in Public Health,
https://doi.org/10.1007/978-3-030-17280-0_11

Table 11.1 Summary of key hazard ratio results for race/Hispanic origin predicting mortality risk with rotating index reference groups

| Variables controlled in analysis | Index reference group | | | | | |
| | Non-Hispanic white | | Hispanic | | African-American | |
	African-American	Hispanic	African-American	Non-Hispanic white	Hispanic	Non-Hispanic white
Year of birth plus…						
Educational attainment	1.35***	0.98	1.37**	1.02	0.73**	0.74***
BMI	1.39***	1.22*	1.14	0.82*	0.88	0.72***
Birthplace region	1.35***	Not applicable	Not applicable	Not applicable	Not applicable	0.74***
Total years played Major League Baseball	1.4***	1.2*	1.17	0.83*	0.86	0.71***
2-way player position	1.45***	1.22*	1.19	0.82*	0.84	0.69***
Handedness (batting)	1.4***	1.2*	1.17	0.83*	0.86	0.72***
All significant variables[a]	1.42***	1.04	1.36*	0.96	0.74*	0.71***

Notes Hazard ratios are for race/Hispanic origin controlling for variables indicated plus year of birth
Hispanic players not included in birthplace region variable
Continuous version of year of birth, BMI and total years played used in all analyses shown
*p < 0.05; **p < 0.01; ***p < 0.001
[a]Includes educational attainment, BMI, total years played, and 2-way position

prediction of mortality risk, above and beyond what race/Hispanic origin explains, none of these items attenuate or otherwise change the relationship between the 2 races.

The empirical results presented in this book are consistent with previously published studies conducted with other groups of former professional athletes like NBA (Lawler et al. 2012; Markowitz 2018) and NFL players (Baron and Rinsky 1994; Baron et al. 2012; Markowitz 2018) that examine mortality risk based on race. The results of the current study provide overwhelming support for the hypothesis that African-American Major League Baseball players have significantly higher all-cause mortality risk than non-Hispanic white players. Even in a special population of professional baseball players, with elevated incomes and high educational attainment relative to the general population, race-related mortality differences are evident.

Based on the data collected in this study, it is impossible to say to what extent, if any, between-race mortality differences among former Major League Baseball players is a function of discrimination, and/or racism that may have been experienced by African-American players, on or off the baseball playing fields. Discrimination and racism are established pathogens for health in general and special populations and their effect on mortality has been well documented in the scientific literature (Williams 2012). "Large, pervasive and persistent racial inequalities exist in the onset, course and outcomes of illness. A comprehensive understanding of the patterning of racial disparities indicates that racism … remains an important determinant" (Williams 2012). Efforts to reduce racial disparities in health and mortality must confront challenges related to discrimination and racism that persist in the US.

This author believes that between-race mortality differences are more social and environmental in origin than genetics-based. There is little doubt that genetic factors play a vital role in health. However, "…they are just one piece of a much larger picture" (Pearce et al. 2004). Few diseases are purely genetic (Lewontin 1993). More commonly, there tends to be interactions between genetics and the environment that influence health and mortality including social, cultural and lifestyle factors. While often difficult to change, modifications of these environmental factors may be required to address between-race mortality differences.

Major League Baseball players, as well as US athletes competing across other professional sports, represent an infinitesimal fraction of the total US population. An argument could be made that the between-race mortality inequalities documented in this book, as well as previously in other scholarly publications, do not represent a major problem because relatively few individuals are affected. However, race-related mortality disparities are a general problem that plague the larger US African-American population. Moreover, while this book has focused exclusively on males, elevated rates of many adverse health outcomes and conditions have similarly been documented among African-American women in the general population that include: breast cancer deaths (Iqbal et al. 2015), pregnancy-complications and maternal deaths (Lu 2018), homicides (Petrosky et al. 2017), stroke (Howard 2013), diabetes (American Diabetes Association 2018), end-stage renal disease (Nicholas et al. 2013), asthma (CDC 2017), hypertension and hypertension-related disease outcomes (Lackland 2014) plus many others.

African-American Major League Baseball players fare much better with respect to mortality than their counterparts in the general population—another finding consistent with several previous studies of professional US athletes (Lawler et al. 2012; Baron and Rinsky 1994; Baron et al. 2012; Markowitz 2018). Collectively, the internal and external findings presented in this book paint a disturbing picture of mortality among African-Americans in the US. Compared to non-Hispanic whites, African-Americans in special as well as general populations are consistently at the low end of the US mortality spectrum.

In general populations, mortality outcomes have improved over time for both races, and encouragingly, the disparities are narrowing. Yet the health and mortality inequalities that persist between the races affect millions of people. Efforts to eliminate race-related health disparities need to be intensified and made priorities in US health and research programs. Given the enduring nature and scope of this problem, it becomes important to approach race-related mortality disparities as a critical societal issue (Williams 2012).

11.1.2   Hispanic Versus African-American Mortality Comparisons

Based on the empirical findings presented in this book, mortality risk comparisons between African-American and Hispanic players indicate a mortality advantage for Hispanics. See the middle columns in Table 11.1 that contain the hazard ratio results between African-American and Hispanic players derived from Cox regressions. With Hispanics as the index reference, the hazard ratios reveal a 12–37% mortality disadvantage for African-Americans. In addition, 2 of the 7 Cox proportional hazards models predicting mortality risk between Hispanics and African-Americans shown in Table 11.1 are statistically significant. While not as robust as the between-race differences, the comparisons between African-Americans and Hispanics provide reasonable support for the hypothesis that Hispanic players have lower mortality risk.

11.1.3   Non-Hispanic White Versus Hispanic Player Mortality Comparisons

In 5 of 7 hazard ratio results between non-Hispanic whites (the index group) and Hispanic players shown in Table 11.1, there is evidence of modest increased mortality risk among Hispanics. The hazard ratio for all of these analyses is about 1.2, or about midway between the hazard ratios for non-Hispanic white players and African-Americans. In the remaining 2 Cox regressions, the only ones containing terms for educational attainment, the hazard ratios for Hispanics are 0.98 and 1.01 reflecting virtually equivalent mortality risk compared to non-Hispanic whites. It is unclear, however, whether the role of educational attainment predicting mortality is real or due to a statistical anomaly. Statistical issues are possible in these comparisons given the relatively small numbers of Hispanic players studied as well as the highly skewed distribution of educational attainment among Hispanics. Strikingly, only 4% of Hispanic players have any college education whatsoever. As a comparison, over 56% of non-Hispanic white players have at least some college education.

11.2 The Hispanic Paradox

In effect, there are 2 different sets of results between non-Hispanic white and Hispanic players with respect to mortality risk depending on whether educational attainment is included in the analyses. When educational attainment is excluded from the analyses, Hispanics have about a 20% increased risk of mortality compared to non-Hispanic whites. When educational attainment is included, the mortality risk between these 2 groups is about the same. The idea that these 2 groups could have roughly equivalent mortality risk is consistent with the possibility of a Hispanic Paradox. Briefly, given substantially lower educational attainment, Hispanics would be expected to have elevated, rather than similar, mortality risk relative to non-Hispanic whites. Additional support for a Hispanic Paradox within the study cohort is derived from post hoc analysis presented in Chap. 9. These results indicate that within Hispanic and non-Hispanic white players with less than a college education, mortality risk among Hispanics is only 8% higher than non-Hispanic white players.

The relatively small number of former Hispanic players in the study cohort increases the likelihood of null results for all paradox-related analyses. In contrast, many of the general population studies demonstrating the existence of the Hispanic Paradox are based on millions of individuals derived from US vital statistics and/or Census data. Larger numbers of players, especially Hispanics, are needed to study this matter further with greater confidence.

It cannot be ruled-out that the finding of similar mortality risk between Hispanics and non-Hispanic whites could be related to the nature of the study cohort; a special population of former Major League Baseball players. In general, players earn more money while playing in the Majors than before initiating their professional careers; they also earn more than their respective general population counterparts. Hispanic cohort players often come from low-income backgrounds and the elevation in their incomes while playing Major League Baseball can be dramatic. Moreover, participation in Major League Baseball since the latter part of the 1960s has featured good health insurance, access to quality health care, and subsequent income from pension and other retirement plans (Major League Baseball Players no date). This income elevation and improved health care access among Hispanic cohort players could help explain their having similar mortality risk relative to non-Hispanic whites. Unfortunately, these mortality benefits do not apply to African-American players.

In several general population studies, a "salmon bias" has been proposed to explain the Hispanic Paradox as a function of the out-migration that generally occurs among older Hispanics. When some out-migrants pass away in their native Latin American countries, death certificates are not registered in the US, deflating death rates and increasing life expectancy among Hispanic residents who do remain. The mortality data on former Major League Baseball players used in the current study are obtained from a sports database that is not reliant on US death certificates. In other words, former players who may have migrated out of the US, and later died in a Latin American country, have a vital status of "deceased" in this study. Consequently, the salmon bias cannot explain the similarities in mortality risk between Hispanics and non-Hispanic whites obtained in the current study.

In addition to the salmon bias, researchers have posited a host of other possible explanations for the Hispanic Paradox (in the general population) like strong social supports (Markides and Eschnach 2005), less cigarette smoking (Fenelon 2013), and selective migration of healthier Hispanics into the US (Palloni and Arias 2004). Another possibility is that there is underreporting of Hispanic origin in US Census denominator counts. To resolve this problem, one research team applied a 7% correction to their data for presumed under-ascertainment of Hispanics (Rosenberg et al. 1999). In the current study, there could be no problem in determining who is Hispanic since this is based solely on their country of origin which is reliably available at sports-reference sites and elsewhere.

Other general population studies that have uncovered a paradox have examined Hispanics who reside in the US. Hispanic cohort players traveled and resided in the US during baseball seasons. However, their off-season residency status during the years they played Major League Baseball is unknown to this researcher.

11.3   Other Independent Risk Factors of Mortality

In addition to race/Hispanic origin, lower educational attainment, overweight BMI, fewer years of playing experience, and playing the pitcher position are independent risk factors for all-cause mortality risk in multivariate analyses that consider all significant variables simultaneously. The following sections discuss the implications of these findings.

11.3.1   Educational Attainment

To my knowledge, this is the first Major League Baseball mortality study that has included a variable that measures educational attainment. The education variable used in this study is a measure developed specifically for this research and its validity is unknown. Given the results of educational attainment analyses documented in this book, it is safe to say that the measure has good "face validity." This is evident, for example, in the results presented in Chaps. 7 and 9 which depict a gradual rise in mortality risk with each successive lower level of educational attainment.

Educational attainment is a critical component of SES. Along with income, occupation and residence, educational attainment is an established predictor of life chances and mortality in special and general populations (Mirowsky and Ross 2003; Zimmerman and Woolf 2014). Educational attainment is generally fixed during the first 2–3 decades of life. However, other elements of SES, like income, can change over the course of a lifetime. This is possibly the case for many Major League Baseball players, particularly African-Americans and Hispanics, who are likely to come from economically tenuous households and communities (Burgos Jr. 2007). Depending on salary level and the number of career years played, the income component of SES can be impacted substantially by participation in a professional US sport, like baseball. Yet the magnitude of the association between education, health and mortality is unknown. In addition, it has proven difficult to tease apart the role of education versus SES aspects like income and occupation (Byhoff et al. 2017). Additional research is required in this area.

Improving educational attainment in any population is likely to enhance health and mortality outcomes. Moreover, since level of education is a modifiable risk factor, it is a prime target for preventative public health efforts that, at least potentially, upgrade both quantity and quality of life. "It [education] influences health in ways that are varied, present at all stages of adult life, cumulative, self-amplifying, and uniformly positive" (Mirowsky and Ross 2003). In addition to health benefits, education can help maximize productivity and income, and may lead to positive economic and social mobility. "Education raises human capital, productivity, incomes, employability, and economic growth. But its benefits go far beyond these monetary gains: education also makes people healthier and gives them more control over their lives" (World Development Report 2018).

The provision of health and nutrition programs in middle childhood and adolescent schools have become ubiquitous on a worldwide basis (Bundy et al. 2016) and can also influence short- and long-term health. For example, school-based immunization programs reach large numbers of students and can include primary and booster vaccinations for health threats like meningitis, measles, hepatitis B, tetanus, and human papillomavirus viruses. Such programs are generally cost-effective and efficacious in preventing morbidity and mortality across large populations of children and adolescents (Ventola 2016). Since effective health intervention programs are infrequently available in poor communities, children attending schools with health programs may benefit the most (Bundy et al. 2016). Hence, in addition to the benefits of education as it relates to improving SES, education may also play a direct role in improving childhood and longer-term health by providing a platform for the delivery of a range of health-related services and treatments.

11.3.2 BMI

Among players in the study cohort, BMI is related to race/Hispanic origin and is also linked to mortality. Furthermore, when BMI is added to the Cox regressions, the association between race/Hispanic origin and mortality is completely unaffected. The results of this study indicate that overweight BMI is an independent risk factor for mortality among former Major League Baseball players, increasing the risk by about 20%.

Overweight and obese BMI levels represent a global public health problem. Unlike the general US population where overweight and obese BMI levels are highly prevalent (National Center for Health Statistics 2018), most professional athletes (except for select weightlifters, wrestlers, football players, etc.) generally have lower BMI scores. Overall mean BMI in this study is 24.6 which is slightly higher than the mean of 23.5 among nearly 1400 NBA players previously studied. The mean BMI of 28.5 among more than 7700 former NFL players is much higher (Markowitz 2018).

According to data compiled by W.H.O., out of 191 countries around the world, in 2016 US adult males have the 11th highest mean BMI (28.8) and rank 11th for the highest prevalence of obese BMIs. More than 72% of male adults in the US have either overweight or obese BMIs (W.H.O. 2016). Given the many documented links between obese BMI and health in general populations, this problem requires serious attention. In at least 2 types of professional athletes, basketball and now baseball players, overweight (rather than obese) BMI levels add to player's mortality risk.

Hispanic players in the current study have significantly lower BMI scores compared to non-Hispanic whites and African-Americans. Less than 27% of Hispanic players have overweight BMIs compared to about 43% in the other 2 groups and mean BMI is almost a full point lower among Hispanics. Of the significant independent predictors of mortality risk, besides race/Hispanic origin and year of birth, i.e., educational attainment, BMI, and playing the pitcher position, only BMI is protective for Hispanics relative to the other 2 groups. These results raise the question whether lower BMI levels among Hispanic players help to offset mortality risk related to low education and player position. Additional research is required to address questions associated with Hispanic origin, BMI and mortality risk.

11.3.3 Pitching

The most surprising finding of the current study is that pitchers are at elevated risk of mortality compared to other player positions. This effect is evident in analyses that control for year of birth alone, as well as multivariate analyses that simultaneously consider all the other significant predictors of mortality. The magnitude of pitchers' mortality risk, while statistically significant, is modest ranging from about 15 to 23%. To my knowledge, no previous mortality research has uncovered an elevated risk for pitchers, although several of the published studies have excluded pitchers. For example, Saint Onge and colleagues (2008) conducted one of the largest life expectancy studies of Major League Baseball players but excluded pitchers stating that: "Our analyses include position players and exclude pitchers due to potential differences in career length and selection into the major league" (Saint Onge et al. 2008). Other baseball researchers, such as Halpern and Coren (1991) and Reynolds (2012) also opted to exclude pitchers from their mortality studies.

In specific sports, such as professional football, player position and body size are strongly related. For example, NFL offensive and defensive linemen have BMIs that average in the obese range, which is significantly higher relative to other position types. While these NFL position categories correlate with mortality risk, once BMI is controlled in multivariate analyses, the effect of position on mortality disappears (Markowitz 2018). In the current study, however, BMI does not offset elevated mortality risk among pitchers.

There is evidence indicating that compared to non-pitchers, pitchers suffer more frequent serious injuries in Major League Baseball that require placement on the Disable List (Posner et al. 2011). However, few if any of these injuries would be considered life-threatening in either the short-or long-term. Given the elevated mortality risk for pitchers uncovered in this study, it would be worthwhile to follow-up with pitchers (and other players) who experience serious injuries during their playing careers to determine whether there is any link with future health and mortality.

Clearly, there is a need to further investigate whether playing the pitcher position is a risk factor for mortality among Major League Baseball players. If current study results are replicated, this would have significant implications for pitchers that would impact on the formulation of preventative strategies going forward. Determining the etiology of elevated mortality risk among pitchers would be critical for constructing successful preventative measures. Players, their representatives, management, owners and other Major League Baseball principals would all have to be involved in addressing this issue.

Unlike several previous Major League Baseball mortality studies, it will be necessary to include pitchers in future research efforts. While there are going to be differences in the number of games played relative to other positions, this can be handled in the statistical analysis. If possible, cause of death data should be collected in future research. Finally, other variables, not captured in the current study, could play a role in the relationship between pitching and mortality. For example, pitchers may have different medical histories or practice life styles that vary from players at non-pitching positions. If possible, additional medical and life style-related data should be collected in future mortality research to determine whether other factors could be accounting for the effect of pitching on mortality risk.

11.3.4 Years of Playing Experience

The current study uncovered several significant results with respect to years of Major League Baseball playing experience and mortality risk. While these results demonstrate an inverse relationship, hazard ratios associated with this effect are modest. A statistically significant inverse relationship between years of playing experience and mortality is reported in at least 1 study of NBA players and a non-significant inverse trend is evident in a study of NFL players (Markowitz 2018).

One thing that is clear from existing studies is that mortality risk does not increase with longer playing careers. Such exposure response effects could conceivably be more likely to occur in a sport like professional football given all the violent physical contact, and long-term injuries including ones involving the head (Mez et al. 2017). Nevertheless, no evidence has been uncovered in previous NFL studies showing a direct effect between length of playing career and all-cause mortality.

The inverse nature of results between years of playing experience and mortality among Major League Baseball players, and others participating in professional sports, may again be related to SES improvements associated with the relatively high salaries earned while playing. Participating in professional sports for 10–15 years or longer can significantly increase players' income and, in turn, lower mortality risk. It is also possible that players who participate in Major League Baseball for longer periods of time have fewer serious injuries which can play a role in long-term health. "Career length is a measure of success and may imply higher levels of physical functioning, motor-skill coordination, talent, and status, which in turn may increase longevity. Players who have long careers might also have better health due to more years of training and support from team physicians" (Saint Onge et al. 2008).

11.4 Other Variables

11.4.1 US Birthplace Region

Because the birthplace region variable used in this study excludes all Hispanic players, analyses of this item are circumscribed. In general, no significant increased mortality risk has been identified, although Major League Baseball players born in the South have a 13% elevated risk in analyses that only control for year of birth. The use of birthplace region in mortality studies of professional athletes is quite limited. In a combined sample of more than 7700 former NBA and NFL players, one study indicates that being born in the Southern part of the US is a significant risk factor for mortality (hazard ratio = 1.35) in multivariate analyses that includes other independent predictors (Markowitz 2018). The 13% increased mortality risk among players born in the South uncovered in this study, while not significant, is directionally consistent with previous limited research in this area.

Based on a variety of economic and social indicators, the South is the poorest and least educated of the 4 US regions. General population death rate and life expectancy data also indicate that the South is the least healthy segment of the US (United Health Foundation 2016). Given these decrements, it is somewhat surprising that birthplace in the South among Major League Baseball players is not a stronger predictor of mortality risk. It must be kept in mind, however, that birthplace region is a crude measure since there is considerable heterogeneity within any region with respect to income, education, residence and other potentially important variables. A player born in the South could be well-educated, wealthy and practice a healthy life style. Additional research is required that uses player-level rather than aggregated statistical data to study characteristics linked to birthplace region as potential predictors of mortality risk.

11.5 Summary and Implications of External Results

Comparisons of mortality rates between professional, elite athletes and various general populations consistently confirm more favorable outcomes for athletes, and the current study is no exception. The external results derived from this study indicate that mortality rates among non-Hispanic white and African-American Major League Baseball players are significantly lower than rates in the general population. A non-significant, directionally consistent trend is also evident among Hispanics. There are several possible reasons that Hispanic players fail to have significantly lower mortality rates than general population Hispanics. First, the sample size for Hispanic players is relatively small. Second, Hispanics in the general population have the highest life expectancy of the 3 groups studied in this book. This could make it more difficult to detect differences with Hispanic players. Finally, the general population mortality statistics are based on Hispanic US residents who may not have been born in Latin America. This differs from the Latin-American born Hispanic players in the study cohort who also may not have resided (year-round) in the US.

The reasons for the mortality rate advantages that have been uncovered among the players are plentiful. As one author puts it: "Major League Baseball players typically have longer life expectancies than the general male population because of their high physical activity and overall health; selection for talent and fitness; favorable heights and weights; low smoking rates; access to high-quality healthcare during their careers; and high prestige and incomes, which allow access to high-quality healthcare during and after their baseball careers" (Saint Onge 2008).

Given the violent and physical nature of professional football, as well as the high prevalence of obese BMIs among these players, the documentation of mortality advantages among NFL players compared to the general population (Baron and Rinsky 1994; Baron et al. 2012; Markowitz 2018; Lehman et al. 2012) are particularly compelling. Despite elevations in neurodegenerative disease mortality risk that includes conditions like dementia, Parkinson's disease, ALS and Alzheimer disease, (Lehman et al. 2012), NFL players have significantly lower overall mortality risk than the general population. If professional football players have lower risk than the general population, it stands to reason that Major League Baseball players, participating in a largely non-violent, much less physical sport with virtually no obese players, would also be advantaged mortality-wise relative to the general population.

11.5.1 Healthy Worker Effect

In general, individuals who are active participants in the workplace are healthier than those who cannot work. The latter group is likely to contain individuals with physical and mental problems that preclude or otherwise limit their employment. In general, Major League Baseball players are not just physically healthy, but are extremely active and fit—at least during their playing days and possibly longer. The healthy worker effect may also help to explain lower mortality rates among Major League Baseball players compared to the general population.

11.5.2 The US General Population: A Low Bar for Comparisons with Professional Athletes

Another key element accounting for significantly lower mortality rates among professional US athletes compared to the general population is the less than optimal state of health and health care in the US. This is reflected by higher mortality rates in the US when compared to rates in other high-income countries and even selected middle-income countries. According to W.H.O., within males there are 36 countries that have longer life expectancies than the US. Males in virtually every Western European country, Australia and New Zealand, Canada, developed Asian countries (i.e., Japan, Israel, South Korea, and Singapore), as well as Bahrain, Cyprus, Qatar, Maldives, Costa Rica, Cuba and Chile all have higher life expectancies than males in the US (World Life Expectancy 2018).

Spending too much on health care and not getting much in return is an unfortunate reality in the US. When comparisons are made with other high-income countries, the US consistently spends the most and has the poorest health outcomes (Schneider et al. 2017). "Based on a broadly inclusive set of performance metrics, …[the] U.S. health care system performance ranks last among 11 high-income countries. The country's performance shortcomings cross several domains of care including Access, Administrative Efficiency, Equity, and Health Care Outcomes..... These results are troubling because the U.S. has the highest per capita health expenditures of any country and devotes a larger percentage of its GDP to health care than any other country" (Schneider et al. 2017).

A plethora of other international health and mortality statistical comparisons, like the ones described earlier in this chapter with respect to BMI, are available that provide further support for the idea that the US general population represents a "low bar" when making comparisons with non-obese, world-class, elite athletes like former Major League Baseball players.

11.6   Study Limitations

This study focused solely on life quantity, which represents only 1 part of a 2-part story. Quality of life data also requires careful examination, when possible, in conjunction with data on life quantity. Since injuries, including ones that result in Disable List placement, are such a common occurrence in Major League Baseball (Posner et al. 2011), longer-term negative health sequalae that impact on quality of life are probable.

In retrospective studies, reliable and valid data should be available that can reasonably address the research questions at hand. As the timeframe covered by a study goes back further in time, obtaining quality data on variables of interest can become increasingly difficult. The current study was dependent on data that covered information that goes back decades. In the case of the oldest members of the study cohort, i.e., players born between 1905 and 1914, some data points go back more than a century. Fortunately, Major League Baseball is a data-rich sport and the Internet provides a platform to obtain reliable and valid data that may not be routinely available for other populations. This is not to say that the data used in this study were easy to obtain. Race and educational attainment stand-out as especially difficult variables to acquire in the current study.

Studies of all-cause mortality are generally worthwhile because rate and risk factor inputs can provide clues for prevention. However, the absence of cause of death data makes it difficult to fully understand how best to reduce risk in vulnerable populations. In combination with more in-depth medical background and life style data, cause of death data can lead to more specific preventative recommendations that may save lives. Nevertheless, the study of all-cause mortality is a useful first step in highlighting areas that require attention in future research efforts.

It has already been mentioned how race is essentially a subjective construct that can be subject to misclassification error. Every effort was been made to identify the race of all US players in the study cohort, but undoubtedly, a small number of individuals have been misidentified. Importantly, there is virtually no error with respect to classifying Hispanic players in this study since this is simply a function of where players are born; a data point very much in the public domain with respect to Major League Baseball players.

Sample size in this study was much larger for non-Hispanic white players relative to African-Americans and Hispanics. This imbalance has the potential to affect statistical results. Moreover, any stratification of the data involving African-American or Hispanic players could be plagued by sparse cell frequencies and lead to uncertain statistical conclusions. Null statistical results, especially, can be due to small sample size and have to be interpreted with special caution.

False positive statistical results associated with the many tests of significance that have been conducted in this study is another limitation. To minimize the likelihood of missing potentially important results, corrections to the alpha level have not been made. Hence, readers are cautioned about the possibility of false positive results reported in this book associated with multiple statistical comparisons.

11.7 Final Comments

Despite its scientific limitations, this study has added to existing knowledge in this important, emotionally-charged, area of inquiry. Mortality research is challenging to conduct even when the individuals being studied are complete strangers. When the deceased are childhood heroes, they become far more than just numbers. Moreover, writing material like this made it impossible to escape thoughts about my own mortality.

Nevertheless, these personal issues have been far outweighed by the insights I've gained while working on this book. The opportunity to be the first researcher to study Hispanic mortality among former Major League Baseball players is an honor for me, especially as the son of parents who grew-up in Cuba. More importantly, the results related to Hispanic players are probably the most interesting ones uncovered in this book and the prospects for future research are vast and exciting.

Results for African-American players represent a replication of previous work in this area. Fortunately, between-race mortality disparities are narrowing in the US general population. Yet, the speed of these changes seems slow and policy-makers must confront these disparities with a rigor and a sense of urgency that is at least commensurate with the underlying problem. In the meantime, public health professionals must continue to identify health and mortality inequities when they exist and work to extend quantity and quality of life, especially for those who are most vulnerable and disadvantaged.

References

American Diabetes Association. (2018). *Statistics about diabetes*. Retrieved from http://www.diabetes.org/diabetes-basics/statistics/.

Baron, S., & Rinsky, R. (1994). *Health hazard evaluation report, National Football League players mortality study*. Report No. HETA 88–085. Atlanta, GA: Centers for Disease Control and Prevention, National Institute for Occupational Safety and Health. Retrieved from http://www.cdc.gov/niosh/pdfs/nflfactsheet.pdf.

Baron, S. L., Hein, M. J., Lehman, E., & Gersic, C. M. (2012). Body mass index, playing position, race, and the cardiovascular mortality of retired professional football players. *American Journal of Cardiology, 109,* 889–896.

Bundy, D. A. P., Schultz, L., Sarr, B., Banham, L., Colenso, P., & Drake, L. (2016). The schools as a platform for addressing health in middle childhood and adolescence. In D. A. P. Bundy, N. de Silva, S. Horton, et al. (Eds.), *Optimizing education outcomes: High return investments in school health for increased participation and learning*. Washington, DC: International Bank for Reconstruction and Development/The World Bank.

Burgos, A., Jr. (2007). *Playing America's game: Baseball, Latinos and the color line*. Berkeley: University of California Press.

Byhoff, E., Hamati, M. C., Power, R., Burgand, S. A., & Chopra, V. (2017). Increasing educational attainment and mortality reduction. *BMC Public Health, 17,* 719.

CDC. (2017). *National health interview survey data 2015*. Table 4-1. Retrieved from http://www.cdc.gov/asthma/nhis/2015/table4-1.htm.

Fenelon, A. (2013). Revisiting the Hispanic paradox in the United States: The role of smoking. *Social Science and Medicine, 82,* 1–9.

Halpern, D. F., & Coren, S. (1991). Handedness and life span. *New England Journal of Medicine, 324,* 998.

Howard, V. J. (2013). Reasons underlying racial differences in stroke incidence and mortality. *Stroke, 44*(6), S126–8.

Iqbal, J., Ginsburg, O., Rochon, P. A., Sun, P., & Narod, S. A. (2015). Differences in breast cancer stage at diagnosis and cancer-specific survival by race and ethnicity in the United States. *JAMA, 313*(2), 165–173.

Lackland, D. T. (2014). Racial differences in hypertension: Implications for high blood pressure management. *American Journal of Medical Sciences, 348*(2), 135–138.

Lawler, T., Lawler, F., Gibson, J., & Murray, R. (2012). Does the African-American-White mortality gap persist after playing professional basketball? A 59-year historical cohort study. *Annals of Epidemiology, 22,* 406–412.

Lehman, E. J., Hein, M. J., Baron, S. L., & Gersic, C. M. (2012). Neurodegenerative causes of death among retired National Football League players. *Neurology, 79,* 1970–1974.

Lewontin, R. C. (1993). *The doctrine of DNA.* London: Penguin.

Lu, M. C. (2018). Reducing maternal mortality in the United States. *JAMA, 320*(12), 1237–1238.

Major League Baseball Players. (no date). *History.* Retrieved from http://www.mlbplayers.com/ViewArticle.dbml?DB_OEM_ID=34000&ATCLID=211157621.

Markides, K. S., & Eschbach, K. (2005). Aging, migration, and mortality: Current status of research on the Hispanic Paradox. *The Journals of Gerontology, Series B, 60*(2), 68–75.

Markowitz, J., S. (2018). *Mortality and its risk factors among professional athletes: A comparison between former NBA and NFL players.* Cham: Springer Nature.

Mez, J., Daneshvar, D. H., Kiernan, P. T., Abdolmohammadi, B., Alvarez, V. E., Huber, B. R., et al. (2017). Clinicopathological evaluation of chronic traumatic encephalopathy in players of American football. *JAMA, 318*(4), 360–370.

Mirowsky J., & Ross C. E. (2003). *Education, social status, and health.* New York: Transaction Publishers.

National Center for Health Statistics. (2018). *Health, United States, 2017: With special feature on mortality.* Table 53. Hyattsville. Retrieved from: https://www.cdc.gov/nchs/data/hus/hus17.pdf.

Nicholas, S. B., Kalantar-Zadeh, K., & Norris, K. C. (2013). Racial disparities in kidney disease outcomes. *Seminars in Nephrology, 33*(5), 409–415.

Palloni, A., & Arias, E. (2004). Paradox lost: Explaining the Hispanic adult mortality advantage. *Demography, 41,* 385–415.

Pearce, N., Foliaki, S., Sporle, A., & Cunningham, C. (2004). Genetics, race, ethnicity, and health. *BMJ, 328*(7447), 1070–1072.

Petrosky, E., Blair, J. M., Betz, C. J., Fowler, K. A., Shane, J., & Lyons, B. H. (2017). Racial and ethnic differences in homicides of adult women and the role of intimate partner violence—United States, 2003–2014. *MMWR, 66*(28), 741–746.

Posner, M., Cameron, K. L., & Moriatis Wolf, J. (2011). Epidemiology of Major League Baseball injuries. *American Journal of Sports Medicine, 39*(8), 1676–1680.

Reynolds R. (2012). Life expectancy and comparative mortality of Major League Baseball players, 1900–1999. *WebmedCentral SPORTS MEDICINE 2012, 3.* Retrieved from https://www.webmedcentral.com/wmcpdf/Article_WMC003380.pdf.

Rosenberg, H. M., Maurer, J. D., Sorlie, P. D., Johnson, N. J., MacDorman, M. F., Hoyert, D. L., et al. (1999). Quality of death rates by race and Hispanic origin. *Vital and Health Statistics, 2,* S68–S75.

Saint Onge, J. M., Rogers, R. G., & Krueger, P. M. (2008). Major League Baseball Players' life expectancies. *Social Science Quarterly, 89*(3), 817–830.

Schneider, E. C., Sarnak, D. O., Squires, D., Shah, A., & Doty, M. M. (2017). *Mirror, Mirror, 2017: International comparison reflects flaws and opportunities for better U.S. health care.* Retrieved from https://www.commonwealthfund.org/sites/default/files/documents/___media_files_publications_fund_report_2017_jul_schneider_mirror_mirror_2017.pdf.

United Health Foundation. (2016). *America's health rankings annual report.* Retrieved from: https://www.americashealthrankings.org/learn/reports/2016-annual-report.

Ventola, C. L. (2016). Immunization in the United States. *Pharmacy & Therapeutics, 41*(7), 426–436.

W.H.O. (2016). *Global Health Observatory (GHO) data: Overweight and obesity.* Retrieved from: https://www.who.int/gho/ncd/risk_factors/overweight/en/.

Williams, D. R. (2012). Miles to go before we sleep: Racial inequalities in health. *Journal of Health and Social Behavior, 53*(3), 279–295.

World Development Report. (2018). *Schooling, learning and the promise of education.* Retrieved from https://openknowledge.worldbank.org/bitstream/handle/10986/28340/9781464810961_Ch01.pdf.

World Life Expectancy. (2018). *World life expectancy map (Male).* Retrieved from https://www.worldlifeexpectancy.com/world-life-expectancy-map-male.

Zimmerman E., & Woolf, S. H. (2014). *Understanding the relationship between education and health.* Institute of Medicine, National Academies Press. Retrieved from https://nam.edu/wp-content/uploads/2015/06/BPH-UnderstandingTheRelationship1.pdf.

Index

Printed in the United States
By Bookmasters